Still in the Mind

*MY MEMORIES OF HELLINGLY HOSPITAL
(1963-1982)*

Elisabeth Gimblett

First published in Great Britain in 2005
by MOONFLOWER BOOKS

British library Cataloguing in Publication Data

Gimblett E.
Title
Still in the Mind
Life stories

ISBN 0-9541438-8-4

Typeset by BlueLight Dataset ©. Hellingly, E.Sussex

Printed and bound in Great Britain by
Antony Rowe Ltd, Eastbourne

UK
This book is printed on acid-free paper responsibly manufactured from sustainable forestry, in
which at least two trees are planted for each one used for paper production.

MOONFLOWER BOOKS ©
PO Box 121. Bexhill TN40 1WA
www.moonflowerbooks.com

CONTENTS

FOREWORD

Some months ago one of my good friends Mary Jo Fanaroff, involved with local history, asked me to jot down my recollections of Hellingly Hospital. I happened to be writing my memoirs and, having just arrived at this period of my life, I decided to revisit it more thoroughly than I would have done otherwise. It was no small task, like trying to disentangle a mesh of multiple threads. It was also very nostalgic revisiting my life at Hellingly. This was a great time and a great place to live and work in. I loved it. I am well aware that anyone could write on the subject and that other people have also a wealth of stories to tell. We all have so much to recall: the good, the bad and the ugly, but more often the very funny...

I have given different names to the patients and I hope I shall be forgiven for the discrepancies you may find in those pages.

I am extremely grateful to Alastair Rennie for his invaluable suggestions in the printing of this book, and for taking on the task. I would also like to thank all the many friends who shared with me their own recollections: Helen Dalton, Mary Jo Fanaroff, Sally Fox, Stephen House, Rita Hopper, Juliette Lusted, Jackie Powell, Nan Sarson (nee Carr), Leone and Brian Scott. Thank you again Jenny, Mary Jo and Sally for proof reading, your suggestions were much appreciated and noted.

I dedicate the memoirs to all the people, colleagues and patients that I have known and cared for over the years I worked at the

5

hospital; who have dropped out, disappeared from my life for some reason or other, but more particularly to Nicole Gwizdeck and Jeannine Harnish Turton, my good friends, who died during the last three years.

Elisabeth Gimblett

October 2004

MY INTRODUCTION TO THE HOSPITAL

For a number of years Matron, Miss Bradley, had placed recruiting adverts in newspapers abroad to get nursing staff, with board and lodgings, monthly wages and the possibility of free training. This made for a very cosmopolitan Hospital, to say the least. Irish nurses were the first to come, then the Scottish, Welsh, Dutch, German, French, West Indians, Norwegians, Filipinos, Mauritians, Spanish, Chinese, etc…(not necessarily in this order) and let's not forget my Canadian friend! There were English nurses at the hospital as well of course, quite a few from the North of England. Nan Sarson who was Assistant Matron in the sixties then Nursing Officer when Matrons were abolished, came from Scotland. She told me that for many years staff had not been allowed to be recruited from the surrounding villages so as not to breach confidentiality.

Having completed three years' training to become a secretary (my father's idea), I was scanning local newspapers for such a job with little enthusiasm. I was not drawn in that direction at all. However when I discovered Miss Bradley's advert I just knew this was what I wanted; it offered adventure, escape from the mundane, mystery, something different definitely. I never thought of it at the time but both my grandmothers had worked in a mental hospital years before; Gabrielle, my maternal grandmother had been an assistant matron on night duty. I had good memories of visiting her as a small child of eight or so. The first time I was in her office she introduced me to some of her patients who made a fuss of me as I was her grand-daughter. I had been enchanted, as I did not usually get that much positive attention! This association must have stayed with me. Another time I enjoyed seeing a play, my first play, performed in the large hall.

I replied to this advert straightaway without telling anyone, and when I was accepted, sprung the news of my impending departure to England to the family. Well, let me tell you, they were delighted; it seemed to me they could not wait to see me go. For the first time in my life my father commended me to my brother and sisters for my initiative. I have to admit a slight sense of dismay as no one said "Don't go darling!" My fate was sealed.

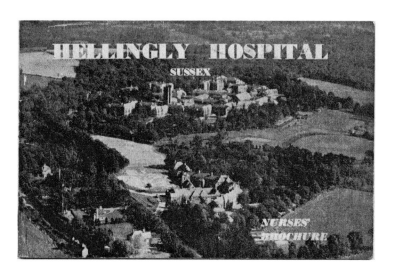

The Nurses Brochure
Sent to me in France October 1963

I travelled to Hellingly via Dover and London; my journey was much longer than it could have been and I missed out on a treat: usually one of the hospital brakes fetched the new French staff arriving at Newhaven, with a friendly nurse and driver to greet them. Anyway, in November 1963 I arrived at Hellingly station, about two years before Mr Beeching disposed of this convenient railway line to Uckfield.

At 8pm, it was already night, pitch-black, and the only person I could ask as to the whereabouts of the hospital was a very shy young man, the only person who alighted from the train with me. I think he was divided by his desire to run away from this outgoing young French girl and good manners to show me the way. The latter won and he walked with me quietly to the cross-roads, pointing me in the right direction. I walked up the drive in the dark with my suitcase, tremulous with excitement, hyped up, but not frightened. It took me a little while to find a door when I came upon Park House. It was the side entrance to the female side. A nurse of about my age came forward to greet me with a smile, asking me my name. I suddenly realised she might think me a new admission, so quickly I told her in my halting English: "I am a new nurse!" Cheerfully the girl gave me a pat on the back and, turning to the sister who was arriving on the scene, told her that I was her friend. For a second I thought this was very odd. I had never met her! I relaxed considerably when she explained she was French as well. (My friend Rita H had a worse experience; she was actually taken to a bed! She was so traumatised she nearly went back to Belgium, where she came from.) Park House being the first building on the drive, it should have been expected that foreign girls would walk in Park House by mistake, come to think of it. The staff should have been aware surely.

Anyway this welcoming girl was allowed to leave work a bit early to take me to the nursing office. While we walked "up the drive" she filled me in the latest happenings: the one that left a mark was that a French girl had died from the gas fire in her room at the nurses' home. No one knew whether she had intended to kill herself, but some thought so. I was a bit perturbed by this,

9

but not overly so; I had so much to take in.

The next day, besides being measured for my uniform, I was taken to the Police station to be issued with a "Certificate of Registration", a working permit allowing me to work at Hellingly Hospital only, according tp the "Aliens Order 1953" This exercise was to be repeated the following year, and in 1967 "the condition attached to the grant of leave to land" was "hereby cancelled". In other words I did not have to report to the authorities any more after this.

My room on the second floor was cosy, a candlewick bedspread covered the bed; there was a chest of drawers with a mirror, a small wardrobe, a chair, a washbasin and mirror, and a rug on the floorboards. Large pipes running through the walls of the nurses' home at the ceiling provided warmth, but there was also the small coin operated and antiquated gas fire; I used that cautiously…

The window looked out on to a courtyard. I remember that on full moon nights, believe it or not, one of the female patients in a nearby ward would shriek and howl. This added atmosphere, shades of Mrs Rochester; it was rather eerie…

On the ground floor by the foyer was a sitting room with a television (it was there that a few days later I saw the news of John Kennedy's assassination). On the whole we met our female friends in our rooms, or we went to the Social Club where we could socialise with men as well. (This club was opened only two months before my arrival, not that I had anything to do with it!). We could use the old common room in the main building if we wanted to hold a party. This is where I met my husband four years later.

We managed surprisingly well without telephones, considering the need for them now. We had the use of a pay phone in the foyer; we used it occasionally, for vital calls. It rang often: if you were a fool like me and picked it up you realised what a nuisance it was… I had to climb up and down the stairs, run around the long corridors on the three floors; often on a wild goose chase. Once I answered a chap from Eastbourne asking for a girl I had never heard of. She might have been a figment of his imagination come to think of it. He said 'Never mind, you sound nice, could you come out and meet me' I did not, if you want to know!

We did not have electric sockets in our rooms then, and if we wanted to listen to our records, or the radio, we had to find the nearest one; in our area we needed a very long extension, running through two long corridors. One evening four or five of us were gathered in Nicole's room , listening to some rather loud and rousing trendy hits while character assassinating her next door neighbour; a girl who had tried to get off with Nicole's husband-to- be. Actually, apart from Nicole, we all knew they had actually done the deed, but we had not told her, as we did not want to shatter her illusions. (Knowing now how her marriage turned out I have often wondered whether it would have been better to let her face reality). Anyway there we were, having a good gossip, making sure the girl heard how we felt about her, when suddenly the music stopped. It turned out this strange girl had cut the electric cable with a pair of scissors! It is a wonder she did not get electrocuted. She got a stiff telling off from the nursing office though, as Nicole reported it straightaway. One of the Assistant Matrons commented that the girl was weird: she had been found dancing in her leotard in the sitting room in the middle of the night apparently (and why not?)

Miss Evans was in charge of the nurses'home. Amongst other things she provided us with clean linen weekly. She inspected our rooms occasionally, when we were not there; she must have gone around each room checking all the beds: she found out that a particular girl had helped herself on a daily basis to clean sheets. (It was such a treat to slip into the freshly laundered and pressed smooth sheets after a hard day's work) She was most indignant this girl had the gall to get into her store cupboard behind her back to help herself. Anyway I remember feeling a bit surprised, as well as privileged, that she shared this bit of information with me. Maybe I was the first person who came along while she was fuming and she had to share her feelings with someone.

The hospital as a community provided all our needs.

There was the large hall at the centre of the hospital, fulfilling different functions. Cinema weekly, Prize-Givings, patients' and staff Christmas dinners, and of course the grand affair of the yearly staff ball which had most of us dressed to the nines and where we, the little people, mingled with the great and the good. Women from the Royal Voluntary Service, (WRVS) used to do occupational therapy in the hall as well. All the patients able to join in would come from the wards. I made a tray and a wastepaper basket there as a student. In the middle sixties qualified Occupational Therapists took over; then a bit later the Industrial Therapy Unit was created in a large prefabricated building, next to Woodside. All kinds of activities were possible there, including filling little bags for Dan Air, with plastic knives, forks and spoons, a serviette, and sugar and salt sachets. (I did that too with our day-patients in Park House in the seventies). This allowed patients to prepare for the routine of work outside the hospital, while gaining some self-esteem and earning a little money.

Across the hall were the hairdresser's and a little newsagent shop, also run by the WRVS. I cannot forget the chocolate bar vending machine, which was a godsend late at night if one was desperate! I often was…

The mess room provided all our meals day and night. The quality of the food was excellent, I think, though I was personally disappointed with my first Christmas pudding and custard, having read Charles Dickens mouth watering account of this feast - the custard was a bit watery. I loved fish and chips but most of all the pies of all descriptions, and the puddings, all this cooked in the great big kitchens. Most of the ingredients came from the hospital farm, vegetable gardens, greenhouses etc. … The milk was taken every morning to Bexhill dairies to come back sterilised the next day. (Years later, in 1969 I travelled back home to Bexhill in this milk lorry. when I worked on night duty).

A small infirmary, with about three beds, opposite Bodiam ward, was used for all kinds of surgical interventions including dentistry until the mid-sixties when the general hospital in Eastbourne took over. Brain surgery had also been performed there well before my time, when that treatment was fashionable. I watched one of the last operations, an appendicectomy, in my first year. Bodiam's ward nurses cared for the sick members of the staff in this infirmary; I looked after Sr. McDonald there when she was very ill. My friend Charlyne had a spell there also, one sunny summer, when she was run over by a motorbike as she was walking along the road to the hospital with her young man. (Matron told her this fellow was not a gentleman or he would have walked on the outside himself!). Anyway for a while, every lunch time, a little band of us, her friends, would cross the lawn with our lunch, from the dining room French windows to the little patio outside the infirmary to keep her company. This was very pleasant, and fun too.

A small room, hidden by the Records office, was allocated to the Roman Catholic worshippers; the Anglicans had a massive red brick Church, with a beautiful rose window. (I understand this window was taken out for safe keeping when the hospital closed)

I confess that I seemed to have forgotten all about my religious duties, what with work and my social life. However Father Brady, the Catholic priest caught up with me in Ditchling ward. He made it his business to know all his flock, of course, and finding out I was French, and Catholic, asked how long I had been at the hospital and why he had not seen me in his services. I told him I usually had to work on Sunday mornings. Anyway the next Sunday blow me if I was not sent on church duty!

The nursing school was a small one-storey building, a prefab, with a classroom and a clinical room.

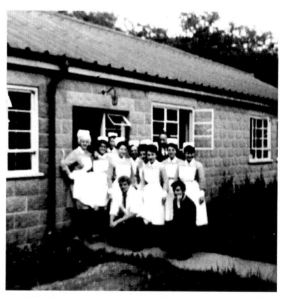

Class February 1964 in front of the school

I started my nursing training in February 1964, three months after my arrival. As we nursed physically ill patients then, up to the late sixties, General Nursing procedures as well as

Psychiatric skills were on the curriculum. Ear syringing, enemas, catheterisations, aseptic dressings, isolation nursing, surgical techniques, etc…(Later students were sent to Princess Alice Hospital for three months experience as well.) We had three tutors, Mr Gutteridge as the Head, Mr Obskarkas and Mr Docherty. I remember because it was explained that their initials formed the mnemonic God or dog… To start with I had to concentrate really hard to understand what was being said. It was easier for me to do the written work. I was pleased when one day Mr. Gutteridge complimented me on my command of the English language: when at a loss I would anglicise French words; these often happen to be unusual English words. However Mr G. rebuked me several months later for not paying attention to what he was saying. In fact I was laughing because my boy-friend could not keep his eyes open, I could see him struggling to do so but not succeeding very well. Watching him made me laugh. He was not caught though, but I was told off for not paying attention! The fact is that by then I could follow a lecture without having to concentrate too much. It has to be said Mr G. had a very soporific voice; slow, deep and monotonous, giving his lecture while walking slowly from side to side of the room in front of us, it was as good as a hypnotherapy session!

I might as well tell you at this juncture that my spoken English was basic. Before my departure from France, I had spent some time with my father, who enjoyed speaking English, working, listening and repeating the very simple, but very correct, Queen's English sentences from the Linguaphone records. I could read and write simple texts but it took me ages to work out what to say, and by the time I could say it, I often found it was too late, the topic of conversation had moved on. (This should have been good training to keep my mouth shut, but I caught up afterwards!). I found everyone speaking too fast for me to understand at first. It must also be said that the different pronunciations, accents, colloquialism and language of patients and staff, who came from all over the world, varied greatly from what I had learnt. I was often surprised to be told the meaning of what I heard ('innit' for instance). It could lead to misunderstanding of course. A few weeks after my arrival, as I was walking along in the corridors with another girl, (I just loved walking up and down those large and gleaming corridors, purposefully, as it always had to be.) a young man accosted me with those words: "Hello luv!"; Flabbergasted I said to my friend: "Honestly, I don't know him!" I thought he was being over friendly, calling me "love"... Another funny thing was that many young men tagged the word "like" after every sentence, even after hello.

Language at the hospital was not often refined, to say the least. I said something to my mother-in-law to be, not long after I met her, prompting her to tell me: "That is not very nice Elisabeth!" I was very quick at picking quaint expressions as well, or clichés, if they were funny to picture, and they are catchy.

Let me tell you about the time a friend of mine, a very pretty French girl, smart and well groomed, got chatted up by several young men in the club, the first time she went there. All attentive, they asked her if she spoke English. She replied: "Oh yes! I can say 'Give me your teef please' and 'sit on the commode'"

There were facilities to take English lessons at the hospital if necessary.

At tea breaks in the winter everyone assembled in the kitchen for a cup of tea, biscuits and a smoke. Anyone could smoke practically anywhere and anytime then; it was often said that it facilitated rapport with the patients, who all seemed to be smokers; they cadged from the staff, so, on two counts, it was good for them. For the first few months I was the only one to refuse cigarettes when they were offered round. I was aware this made me feel unsociable, so I decided to take up the habit;

besides I had been told that if you stopped smoking you put on weight, so I figured if I started I would lose it! It worked, but only because I replaced a meal with a glass of milk and a cigarette; for a short while, I hasten to add! Then years later, in the seventies I suddenly noticed I was the only smoker in a meeting. I had become anti-social again, and even more so. I started thinking of giving it up. That was not so easy.

Opposite the school was another small prefab. The "isolation" ward was for three or four patients who were typhoid carriers and not allowed out. There was only one nurse per shift and so three nurses were their only contact with the outside world. They had a television, and were able to walk and garden in the area surrounding the building, looking over the South Downs, so at least they had a view. I never worked there, but Jackie remembers the rules surrounding the disinfecting of every item used. Apparently these patients were transferred to another hospital at a later stage.

In the late seventies I think, these prefab buildings gave way to the Secure Unit and a car park...

Matron, Miss Bradley, had a small office next to Bodiam ward, opposite the infirmary. She was exactly as most people imagine a matron to be: formidable, tall, large, well cushioned, and solid looking. She was down to earth, no nonsense, and fair, with a warm sense of humour. I think everyone respected and trusted her, and many liked her. I did, very much, though she frightened me a little. (She reminded me of my grandmother!) Her uniform consisted of a thick navy blue dress with a soft white collar, a little frilly white cap, and, like the rest of us, she wore black tights and black lace-up brogues. I cannot remember her out of uniform, ever. She lived on her own, in a flat, next to the nurses'

17

home. She kept her ear to the ground and seemed to know everything; she occasionally raided the nurses'home, because she heard a rumpus no doubt.

She would see and welcome the new staff, individually, or in small groups of two or three, depending on the arrivals I suppose, and give us a talk about her expectations, our duties and what was not on. When I first heard from her, a few days after my arrival, that we were not to go to the male block I was shocked… because I had never considered such a dreadful thing! And only a month later I was faced with this opportunity…Well, it was Christmas and we were invited to a party…

Though some said Matron could understand French, she always asked someone to interpret for her, as few French girls could understand English when they started, let alone speak it. I was particularly proud the first time I was called to translate for her within my first year.

❦

MATRON'S INTRODUCTORY LETTER TO FRENCH NURSES
(Translated from the French by myself.)

DAILY ROUTINE

Morning shift

6am   wake up call by the night staff

6.30-7am   breakfast

7am to 2pm time on duty

2 pm   lunch

Afternoon shift

8.30am   breakfast

midday   lunch

1pm to 9pm time on duty (teatime as arranged by the Charge Nurse)

9pm   supper

Meal times when off duty

8.30am   breakfast

12am to 1pm lunch

4pm to 4.30   tea

7pm   supper

When you are off duty and want to have your supper later you have to arrange this in the morning with the mess room staff.

LAUNDRY

Soiled uniform must be taken to the laundry room Friday, no later than 3pm.

Clean uniform must be fetched from the laundry the following Thursday.

Change of sheets and towels

Sheets and towels must be exchanged for clean ones every Wednesday or Thursday in the Nurses home Sister's office.

BEDROOMS

Beds must be made before going to work.

Bedrooms must be clean and tidy.

Keep your bedroom well ventilated.

Sleep with your window open.

Switch the gas off before going to bed.

Uniforms out of use or needing repair must be taken to the sewing room on Mondays or Tuesdays each week.

KEYS

All keys must be left with the head porter each time you leave the hospital.

SEWING MACHINES AND DRYERS can be borrowed on demand from the nursing home's Sister.

NURSES' HOME

You are not allowed to invite men to the Nurses'home, or to go to theirs.

G. M. BRADLEY, MATRON

Matron came to the school occasionally for one reason or another, but always gave a talk to each new intake of students. Again it was about her expectations; that everything we did in or out of the hospital reflected on the good name of the Hospital so at all times we should behave appropriately. She demanded from us kindness, compassion, thoughtfulness and dedication to the patients. She told our group of her visit to a friend who was recovering from an operation in a general hospital. This lady was very weak and had been unable to get to the food a nurse had placed on the table at the end of her bed; another nurse came back a while later to pick up the plate which clearly had not been touched. The patient had gone on without food. Recalling this story Matron was visibly upset by this lack of care and neglect; she was very forceful in letting us know that if she ever found out such a thing had gone on in her hospital the culprit would be out.

Dr. Rice, the Medical Superintendent, the big chief, also visited us at the school. He gave us a terrifying lecture on venereal disease, its history and consequences. This was no doubt intended to keep ourselves to ourselves, as people used to say. The pictures he projected still come back to mind...There were still a few patients in the hospital with GPI, the third and final stage of syphilis. You might be better dead...

Men were paid weekly, female monthly (maybe it was thought we were better at budgeting!) We queued in the corridor, at the Pay Office and through a little window we were handed our pay packet to sign for, a little brown envelope containing cash. My first pay was £18. Sometime later cheques were deposited in our bank accounts for security reasons. The Pay Office also dealt with patients' DHSS monies. Initially, in geriatric wards, or in wards where people were severely disturbed, this money would be entrusted to the Charge nurses or Sisters to dispose of according to the various needs of the patients. Chits had to be signed by the staff and a full account of expenses recorded. After1967 all money given to the patients able to handle it, had to be collected and signed for by the patients themselves, and chits handed to the pay office. This was prompted by the discovery that two Charge Nurses asked some patients to hand their money for "safe keeping", and pocketed it themselves... They were found out. One managed to escape retribution by doing a bunk, taking with him at the same time a hoard of electric equipment that he had accumulated over the years in the store cupboard. For good measure, at the same time he also went off with the sister on the opposite shift.

When the hospital started discharging patients into the community I know of at least one elderly canny patient who had saved all his money, something like several thousands pounds, after decades in the hospital. He was not happy to leave, the hospital was his home and he would have to start spending his own money from then on. Of course; he was not entitled to further aid, he was a rich man.

Also in the main building, was the Pathological Laboratory, with the nice "blood ladies" (phlebotomists) calling round the wards to take blood samples for clinical investigations carried out at Hellingly until the late seventies. There were also the Radiotherapy department, the Works department, the sewing room, laundry, upholsterers, porters galore, the tailor, the tinker, the candlestick maker no doubt, and please forgive me for forgetting a few, as I am sure I have. I expect others will pop up as I describe life on the wards. Believe me, I am not embellishing anything when I tell you all these good people were friendly and chatty, ready to help, and the morale was good overall.

The consultants, social workers and psychologists had their offices in Woodside. Also in Woodside, Mr Lindfield was the man in charge of the records department. With its thousands and thousands of patients' records and ledgers it was nevertheless possible to obtain files and information very quickly. I am not sure that computers are as efficient now as Mr Lindfield was then, in his access, organisation and memory - I am not blaming the computers you understand - besides he was always courteous and a very interesting person to talk to.

As in any other hospital, someone had to tell you sooner or ter that the tower was to incinerate dead bodies; it sounded much more interesting than a plain old water-tower. As for the mortuary, you were often told with glee that someone or other had been locked in the frozen compartment. I dare say it might have happened at least once!

Finally, to cap it all were those magnificent grounds, kept to perfection by the Head Gardner, the gentle and unassuming Mr Luscombe and his team, all beavering away everywhere; to delight the eyes and the senses, provide peace and the joy of nature; parks, and lawns, flower beds, bushes galore, meandering paths through ancient and newly planted trees, leading to clearings in the woods looking over the South Downs in the distance, where I would read a book on a sunny afternoon and relax. All this was ours. There was a tennis court for staff and patients, which one of the doctors' wives would use with her friends occasionally, to our annoyance as she had a perfectly good one in her own spacious garden! The football pitch held no interest for me but the cricket field did, with its pristine lawn. The smell of freshly mown grass was an overwhelming new sensation, my first spring in England; there is nothing like the smell of an English lawn after the cut! Lawns in France are few and mangy, and you are not allowed to walk on them. Many of us girls often rolled down the steep banks of this cricket pitch, at dusk, when no one else was likely to see us! We felt wonderfully silly!

It was usually before or after an exam, when we were likely to be a bit tense, that we were allocated to go out with a Social Worker or the Welfare Officer, as it was known to be a care-free day. So it was in my third English summer that I went visiting patients with them. I cannot remember much of the Welfare Officer's role. It related to patients' finances I think. However I was very impressed with the Social Worker, Miss Nanny; her name was very suitable; she was lovely, caring, efficient and knowledgeable. Social Workers were primarily concerned with the practicalities of a patient's home life before discharge: children, income, work, housing, etc. They helped in all manner of ways, then they would follow the patients up after discharge until they were satisfied the patients were able to function independently. I read once this little story: a man, walking on the moors, falls in a deep hole; he is stuck, cannot get out; he cries out "Help!" A counsellor happens to pass by. She/he asks, very concerned: "Do you want to tell me how you got in this hole? It must be difficult for you there. How do you feel being in this hole? Have you thought how you are going to get out of this hole?" And then another person passes by; "Hi mate, Here's a rope!"… Which would you prefer in a fix?

As part of my training I made various visits : Roffey Park Clinic was at the height of modern thinking in the sixties, using LSD treatment; controversial even then. We were shown the room where patients were left to their own devices, under discreet observation, (I think there may have been cameras on the ceiling) with different materials, like paints and crayons, under the influence of the substance, to draw or paint, and rant and rave. All their activities and hallucinations were later explored and analysed in depth to unravel their psyche. We were overawed but far from convinced of it as a suitable treatment, let me tell you.

Other visits were to Laughton Lodge and Leybourne Grange, for patients with Learning disabilities, an observation ward in Brighton General, a Child Guidance clinic in Hove, a "remand" home, a resettlement training centre in Leatherhead, and in Hailsham a youth club and the Old Companions Club. Don't think I have a good memory, I am reading my Record book.

SECURITY

Dr Rice had the front gates removed and instigated the open door policy at Hellingly when he took over in the mid fifties. He was particularly proud of it, and we were often reminded how great it was. He would do his rounds, day or night, querying any locked doors. However we did have to have our female or male master key with us, as many parts of the hospital still had to be locked, all back doors certainly. Each ward had to review the policy according to the current situation.

Padded rooms had been condemned before my time, apart for one or two used as a show case or museum. The museum in Park House was enlightening to visit: there were huge admission ledgers, with patients' records and their photos, on admission and discharge. I was interested to notice they usually looked cheerful on arrival but most miserable on discharge.

The side rooms served different purposes in every ward. Some were used for physically ill patients, some for patients who had recovered and could have their privacy, and some for disturbed patients. In the latter case a nurse would stay in with the patient at all times, the door being left open. Some of these doors were self-locking, if I remember rightly, and you could not use a key on the inside. I was sitting next to a bedridden and unpredictable patient in Fairlight ward one lunch time, when somehow the door was shut on us. Help! I thought. I did not want to cause a fuss and upset the patient, who was oblivious to what was going on; I pretended to be calm while I was frantic. However I was eventually able to call to another nurse in the dormitory through the small window in the door, and pretty soon she rescued me.

Many wards had a special patient; usually someone who had recovered from their mental illness and seemed with it and capable, even if a little eccentric sometimes. They had been in the hospital for so long it was their home, and it would have been thought cruel in those days to discharge them to outside life where they had no one. These patients also had their own side rooms. They often took on a helper's role; they worked in the wards, or Industrial therapy, or even outside the hospital. Others would carry out tasks like making the tea, sandwiches or toast for the staff breakfast, or report on things they found untoward, even supervise the staff when the charge nurse was off. In Guestling ward in the late sixties, "old Joe" told me that the Charge Nurse would not approve of what I was doing, as it was not his way; a trained staff nurse by then, I considered my method more suitable than this particular Charge Nurse's, known to cut corners in many areas. I told Joe it may be so but I happened to be in charge that day, so that was that!

In Arlington ward there was a dear old thing who used to make superb toast for our elevenses. She kept them hot for us, in a plate over a bowl of boiling water. At some point she must have thought Sister White was below par and not very happy;

she crushed her own anti-depressant tablets and put them in Sister'sandwiches, (how long for we do not know)...Eventually she was caught doing it, and this was the end of the sandwich making! The story did not say if Sister improved with her treatment...

I think it was in the early seventies that a few elderly wanderers, having got lost in the woods, prompted the fitting of special handles on the doors, placed in such a way both hands were needed to open them. Patients with dementia could not work them out apparently.

Mr Gutteridge, our head tutor, told us a story of a man who came to the hospital for a job as a gardener in the old days. He got lost in a corridor and caught up in a crocodile of patients walking back to their ward. Before he knew what was going on he was counted in! The attendant, as they used to be called, could not understand how he had acquired another patient but would not believe the chap, who was in a real panic by then. Happily the charge nurse intervened and freed our man. He went straight home and did not apply for the job after that, surprise, surprise...

I have often pondered in the last ten years about the way doors were locked to keep the patients in before the fifties, and how gradually this has changed to them being locked and secured, by very sophisticated means, to keep the patients out! Up to the nineties office doors were open to everyone practically all the time, unless there was a meeting or conference in progress. There was always a member of staff available there. Patients could, and would, wander in the office and have chats with the staff. The small offices often had only one desk, for the sister or the charge nurse. As a staff-Nurse, I walked in Park House office once, to find our gay, witty and very popular Charge Nurse B. being chased by a playful young girl, a patient who seemed to be trying to kiss him, as he was trying in vain to wave her away with his arms. I was amused by this comic scene but came to the rescue by shooing her out: "Leave the man alone!" said I. After she walked out with a giggle, B. looking a bit discomfited to be caught in such a flurry, told me "she was not trying to kiss me, she was smelling my after-shave! Its called 'Brute'!" This was the cherry on the cake as far as I was concerned.

Staff nurses and student nurses would frequently walk in to write notes or report something, but usually most of us were about our jobs with the patients. It was a constant refrain, instilled from the start, and repeated again and again "Go and talk to the patients". The situation is now such, in some cases, that sometimes the entire staff is behind locked doors. Sad to say much has changed to accommodate all the paperwork linked with both statistics, and covering us for fear of litigation.

STAFF

The hospital served three different areas, Eastbourne, Hastings Bexhill and Rother, and Tunbridge Wells. All staff worked throughout the whole of the hospital until the early seventies when we were separated in these three areas. There was a sense of the family having broken down, strange as it may seem. We lost touch with people we had enjoyed working with.

Overseeing all was Dr David Rice. He lived with his family at Bow Hill, a large mansion with a spacious garden and a tennis court, now housing the Mental Health Administration and their car park. I have a very hazy concept of what the Hailsham Hospital Management Committee did. As far as I am aware there was only one administrator in the early sixties, and we rarely saw him but at the Prize giving. Most of the Consultants psychiatrists and registrars lived on the premises, in villas or flats. They often asked us nurses to baby sit. We were quite happy to do so: they and their wives were pleasant and friendly, the children rarely any trouble, and we were always offered a nice little collation in their living room, a chat and always some money on our way out. We enjoyed baby sitting for them and most of us refused to be paid. There was only one doctor however who seemed to take it for granted we were there for his family's convenience. He never asked us himself but arranged for one of the assistant matrons to get one of us minions to baby-sit, usually at short notice. It was difficult to refuse, and then nothing was ever offered at the end of the evening.

Miss Bradley was the Matron and Mr Thompson the Chief Male Nurse, until he retired in 1965. Then Miss Bradley became Principal Nursing Officer, with Mr Hard as her deputy. However she was still Matron to us… All her Assistants, female and male became Nursing Officers, and slowly nursing staff also became integrated, in ranking order.

The protocol was strict regarding the uniform, particularly for the women. The male staff all wore grey suits, white shirts and tie, and a white coat on duty.

Women (nor men, but at the time it was hardly likely to be in question!) were not allowed make up or jewellery, and long hair had to be up. We had to be correct at all times out of respect for the patients and so we could not offend anyone. How we would have reacted to find future nurses would expose their belly buttons over jeans and under skimpy tops for all to see I cannot imagine! Work was not a market place where we were on show.

Assistant-matrons wore green dresses with a little non-starched collar and a little frilly white cap like Matron.

Sisters wore navy dresses, white aprons, black belts and silver buckles, which they bought for themselves when they had passed their final exam, were registered with the General Nursing Council and become Staff Nurses. They wore large starched caps, floating like a galleon on top of their heads - Believe me it often looked like that when with-it young Sisters back-combed their hair as high as it could go!.

Two ward sisters were in charge of the whole ward management until the seventies when the domestic services branched out with their own managers. This frequently caused problems as they had different directives and goals... Should anything unusual need sorting out in the domestic area, Sister had to contact the supervisor to negotiate a satisfactory outcome to the situation. That person, not based on the ward, might be unavailable so the ward had to wait for action. In Park House we were told that it was difficult for them to do whatever was asked for, as "we have to work around the tea breaks"! Never mind, it is even crazier now...

Somehow, in most wards you had the "good" (friendly) sister and the "bad" (frightening) Sister. Shifts are necessary but can create problems as well. Both shifts meet for the hand-over at lunch-time. In the sixties the sisters, on their own, would discuss the agenda for the day and any problems. Later, sometime in the seventies, the whole staff, or practically the whole staff, would assemble and participate. My experience was that, often, they chose that time to blame the night staff for anything amiss, and after the meeting, when the staff from the previous shift had gone, they would blame them. I noticed this as I had the dubious privilege to work across shifts. The night staff did not blame anyone as far as I can remember.

Seconding the sister was a staff nurse, who wore a thick denim-like material grey dress, a stretchy belt and silver buckle, or a SEN (State Enrolled Nurse) whose dresses and belts were green. Student nurses and auxiliaries wore pale blue dresses with white belts.

Prior to 1965 SENs used to gain their title in recognition of several years of auxiliary experience and they deferred to first year students. Then they were required to train for a year to receive this particular grade when they became able to take precedence over first year students.

At the end of their first year, student nurses had to pass the "Prelim" exam in order to continue with their training, and then they were given a dark blue starched belt to wear. Student Nurses were part of the work force, "hands on", as it is said now, and by their third year they were able to run a ward efficiently and confidently. Should they need help they knew they could always telephone the Nursing Office where they would find support and guidance twenty four hours a day. (Even with mobiles you don't get that in the Community)

We all had to wear sturdy shoes and black tights. One day as I was passing Matron's office when she happened to be sweeping her doorstep, she noticed my stockings were not as they should have been. She pointed this out to me: "Nurse, those stockings are brown!" I told her I had been sold them as black. "Then you've been diddled!" she said with good humour.

We wore a clean apron every day, and a little starched cap on our heads. I must not forget the stiff starched collar, attached with studs, which cut into my neck, and the cuffs. These cuffs, equally starched and attached with studs, had to be on and off the whole shift. You arrived on a geriatric ward with them on; you took them off and rolled up your sleeves to get the patients up, to toilet, wash or bathe them, lay the tables, take them to the tables, make the beds, and indeed to fulfil any task. You had to have your cuffs back on to serve the food, give medication, at quiet times, and when visitors called. Usually these visits were unexpected. So, if you were in the middle of something, as quickly as possible you rolled your sleeves down and put the cuffs back on. This could be quite a performance.

Many of us found it difficult to be always spick and span! For instance, once we were in the dormitory when we heard Matron was on her way. I knew I looked a complete disaster, probably egg on my apron, cap askew and hair dishevelled. I did not want her to see me like that so I put the curtains round a bed and hid there, praying she would not walk in. She did not.

One of my friends, L., as a young student nurse, was caught without her cap on, as a disturbed patient, assaulting her, had just knocked it off her head. The assistant matron walked in on the scene, saw what was going on, but reprimanded the nurse for being bare headed.

I must not forget our cape, large and capacious, to keep us warm outside, and when on night duty. It was made in a very thick woollen navy blue material, lined red, with 2 long red ties crossing over the chest and buttoning behind. We all loved it. I kept mine for years as a souvenir when the uniforms were abandoned in the middle seventies. It eventually became moth eaten and I had to throw it away.

Uniforms gave us a kind of protection, a status, a certain confidence, when we were young.

When we were on the morning shift one of the night nurses on their rounds gave us our wake up call, banging on our door, where we had left a note for her to do so, shouting "6 o'clock!". I never managed to get enough time for breakfast before 7am, so I was famished by the time we had got the patients up, washed and fed. I used to put a leftover hard-boiled egg in my pocket, from the patient's breakfast, and eat it later. Of course by that time the shell was crumbling away, and it was disgusting (sophisticated I never have been!).This was strictly against the rules; all left over food was to go to the hospital farm in huge refuse bins, but I figured the pigs would not miss it. We used to have a small break, with a cup of tea, biscuits, or toasts in some wards, for our elevenses; I was starving by then.

If you lived in you were more likely to be asked to do another shift should there be staff shortages. We could even be asked in the morning if we could work that same night, or do a long day. A few nurses volunteered for long days as this would make extra money or time in lieu. The work in a geriatric ward is physically tough, from 7am to 9pm. We had to do a spell on night duty at least once a year.

In the early sixties the Domestic staff did not work at the weekends. So then the junior staff, including first year student nurses, would be employed vacuuming, washing, waxing and polishing the floorboards. I remember it well in Bodiam ward sitting/dining room. The patients, tables and chairs would be carried or pushed to one side of the room so we could clean the other side. When this was accomplished we would transport the patients and furniture back to the clean side and proceed with the dirty one. This was done with much goodwill, energy and fun. I cannot remember anyone in those early days complaining that whatever we were doing was not a nurse's job. This came about when males came to work with females. Indeed we women did all manner of work without batting an eyelid, and took it all in our stride, as part of nursing care.

WARD EXPERIENCES

Each ward catered for a particular patient group. These were, and I quote from my booklet entitled "Record of Practical Instruction",   several "Admissions", "Psycho-neurotic", "Acutely sick", "Disturbed", "Epileptic", "Convalescent", "Chronic patients", "Geriatric and infirm" wards. . These last two kinds of wards did not usually have student nurses.

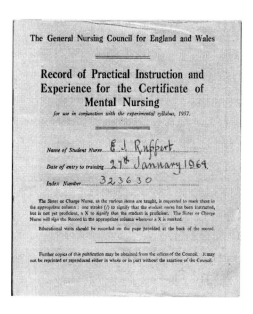

I was first warded in Cuckfield, a geriatric ward, and started on the afternoon shift. I was only there for around two months, give or take one or two exceptions, until I commenced my nursing training.

I remember first being very impressed by some of the old ladies, looking very dignified and ladylike. It was the policy in those days to keep people's hair in their own style to allow them individuality. So long hair was not cut. Besides, it allowed beneficial contact between patient and nurse; contact, touch, closeness with others is an important basic need which patients in hospital often lack. I enjoyed brushing and making their hairdos, and hopefully they enjoyed it too! A few years later, coming back to work on a geriatric ward after some time away, I noticed that most of the patients had the same hair cut, short and practical for the staff no doubt, or for the hairdresser who came around the wards. Like our cells, but much faster than every seven years, policies change…

At meal times porters brought round great big heavy trolleys loaded with food in large containers. The nursing staff then lifted these containers to place them all on the kitchen table, ready to be served by both Sisters when they came back from "handing over". The Sisters then passed the plates with food through the hatch to the nurses in the dining room, to be distributed to the patients. It was in my first few days there that, wanting to be of use, I decided to pick up the container of peas from the trolley… and dropped the whole thing on the floor! Panic, pandemonium, hot and cold sweats for me, but all the staff rallied around. We saved the top layer of peas and scooped up the rest to throw it in the bins and the lit fireplace (the smoke was terrible…). By the time the sisters arrived on the scene the situation was restored. However I could not believe that no one would tell on me, or that one of the sisters would not notice some of the green peas stuck between the floorboards. I was terrified. Sr. T. was absolutely ranting that only a handful of peas had been sent for thirty or so patients. She telephoned to the kitchen straightaway to complain and asked for further supplies immediately. No one told on me…I did not have it in me in those days to own up. I told Sr Sinnot forty years later, at our centenary reunion. She laughed and said "poor kitchen staff, taking the blame!"

I learnt one of the most important lessons, and not just for my nursing role, on my first hour, in Cuckfield. It was mealtime; everyone was sitting down at the table, their meal in front of them. One lady, with patrician features, very regal, hair up in a chignon, just sat there, looking into the distance, unaware of her food. Of course I did what came naturally. I went to her, took her spoon and was just about to feed her when all the staff was on top of me! "Don't!" Well I was stumped! Then they told me. If I fed her she would lose her ability to feed herself. All I had to do was put the spoon or fork in her hand...

I was told how to make a perfect bed. Two nurses were needed, one at either side of the bed. We placed a chair at the foot of the bed to receive the sheets and blankets which we folded down one by one, and replaced in the same manner, making sure each layer was spot on; the corners were important. (Some of us still make beds like this at home, including my sister in France!) With two people it was easy, and could even be enjoyable, like a rhythmic dance. However on a few occasions we were short of staff and had to do the job on our own. One such day I was doing my best, but impatient I made a few beds quickly, without following the correct procedures. Then I saw Miss Grant and another assistant matron walking down the corridor towards the dormitory where I was. I immediately reverted to run around the bed, etc. "Good morning Nurse" said she, and me "Good morning Miss Grant" with a little nod of my head towards her. And then I heard her say to her colleague, amused: "Look at this little nurse, making the beds properly on her own!" So I resumed making the beds the easier way!

I also learnt some more basic English within a week. There was an SEN on that ward, I recollect her walking with a kitchen towel in her hand, looking busy; she was a prototype for others I saw through my career...Very soon I had caught on that the ones who usually did the least had the knack of looking important, walking everywhere as on a mission, as we say now, and a kitchen towel was as good as anything... She stopped me doing whatever I was doing to tell me curtly to go and clean the faeces in the toilets. (Domestic staff has never been allowed to deal with patients' bodily fluids) Now, as it happened, I had never heard of the word "faeces"...It is not usually one you are taught as a French schoolgirl! Bemused, I said "sorry?" she repeated her words once or twice, then getting cross, seeing I still did not have a clue, or may be thinking I was pretending not to, she shouted the four-letter word in my face. I understood then, and laughed, and did as she said. This incident reinforced the need for me to do my nursing training... I did not want to be bullied by people like her, or to have to clean the loos... though I can't help thinking that I probably did equally unpleasant tasks during my training!.

Within my first month I was sent to Ditchling Ward, in the afternoon. There must have been a severe shortage of staff as Sister was by herself when I arrived. The ward was for "disturbed" patients, and everyone had warned me about it. Sister, a pretty, lively young woman, very likeable, explained the patients were mostly what used to be called "subnormal" then, but not all. One had General Paralysis of the Insane, at the third stage of Syphilis; she was very unpleasant at the best of time. We were told it was part of the illness, however this could be reinforced by the fact that few liked to come near her because they feared her nasty responses. All patients showed signs of severe mental impairment of some kind. Most had been there forever, since the thirties possibly. One particular woman had been "committed" to the Hospital since she had had a baby outside of marriage, decades ago. After this she had become mute, withdrawn, and out of touch with her environment. In the mid-fifties after Dr Rice took over, everyone's IQs were assessed, and they found this lady had normal intelligence, no learning disability at all. With encouragement, by the time I saw her she had become slightly more communicative, even if monosyllabic, and was able to participate in some light day-to-day activities. She was an intensive and compulsive knitter.

Then Sister warned me about the two most violent women there, and how to calm them down. One had been diagnosed as an "Idiot". She was short, very stocky and strong as an ox; she had killed someone years ago, before coming to Hellingly. She would seem all right but suddenly she would launch herself at you, screaming, as to attack you. In order to calm her down you had to slap her hand, and that usually did the trick. If not she had to be taken to her side room, the door of which was self-locking. She was not to be detained for more than half an hour. As for the other dangerous patient, she was one of those everyone who met her cannot help but remember. She scared most of us. H., a great big towering woman, (and I am only 5 foot), had also killed someone. Now to restore her good mood if she became agitated, we had to sing to her "Ramona"... A few minutes after this introduction Sister told me she was going next door for a few minutes. She would not be long. She left me on my own, in the sitting room, behind closed doors, with thirty or so weird and crazy people. Being very new I did not think I could just step out and sit in the dining room, next door, where I could still have seen the patients through the glass partition. Some of the patients were sitting quietly staring into space, our friend was knitting furiously, some were rocking to and fro, but the majority were milling about that room, some muttering, some shrieking, or laughing wildly. I was absolutely terrified! And then, several times running, the "Idiot" dashed towards me from one end of the room, screaming; I slapped her hand, she went away, and then it was H. marching down slowly to stand over me, with an evil smile (which comes to my mind's eye straight away!) and I tried to sing "Ramona", quivering "Ramona, lalalalala", as I knew the tune but not the words in English! She seemed pacified for a while afterwards, but then came back for more. Come to think of it she must really have enjoyed my performance; it must have been a novelty for her....

I still cannot believe this time lasted only a few minutes. They seemed like hours...Was I glad when Sister came back! The relief of seeing her was so overwhelming I could not show her any resentment for having been left in this bedlam. It did make me realise how any sane person could become mentally ill if confined there for more than a day, with no possibility of getting out, not being listened to, not heard, not acknowledged. At least I knew there was to be an end to my trial. I certainly felt for the poor woman who had been incarcerated there years ago because she had a baby out of wedlock.

By the time I came back to Ditchling several months later, a great number of patients had been transferred to Laughton Lodge when it was decided that "Learning Disability" was to branch out as a separate speciality. Ditchling now cared for epileptic patients and psychopathic personalities, the bright, the not so bright, the young and the old. This mix was not healthy. Over the years the term "psychopathic personality" seems to have disappeared from the nursing vocabulary, along with other words, discreetly discarded, which have become unmentionable, not Politically Correct. Others have come to replace them and they will be discarded eventually as well.

Most of the patients slept in a large dormitory, at a guess about thirty beds. In the middle sixties it was decided to create partitions with fitted wardrobes/lockers, between each bed, to create a kind of cubicle for privacy. The intention was no doubt very good but I was not that keen. It made the north side of the dormitory very dark during the day and difficult for observation at night; a bit creepy, and it was hard to know which bed to go to if we heard a noise, such as someone having a fit. We had torches but they could wake patients so I did not usually switch it on.

It could be difficult sometime to assess what kind of fit a patient was experiencing, (epileptic, hysterical, or malingering). One of the pay-offs for one particular patient, expert at mimicking fits, was the drug she was given to stop what we thought was "status epilepticus", (continuous fits over several minutes.) The other pay off was the nursing care, the solicitude and human touch.

Even in those days I wondered why some patients were in hospital. The young and the bright were complicated personalities; they would have been better seeing therapists individually or in family units, with specially trained staff.

One girl, we'll call her D, who must have been in her late teens, or just about twenty, should not have been in that ward, learning unhealthy coping mechanisms from hardened institutionalised patients. One of my colleagues, M, told me how once, in the early sixties, when she was left in charge of the ward for half an hour, at tea time, she had done something which plagued her for years. She had been faced with that young girl, D, having a screaming fit in the dormitory, for no reason she could fathom. M, around the same age as the girl, was nonplussed. All she could do to start with was to stare at D. shouting at the top of her voice only occasionally stopping for breath. A bunch of patients had assembled around both of them, very interested to know how the situation would develop, giving her advice. Aware of the excitement reinforcing the problem, M. told them all to get back to the sitting room; which they did, without trouble. She was surprised about that, her first command obeyed. Then facing D, who was still shrieking totally out of control, M. slapped her face. She said she did not know what came over her, but afterwards she remembered this was the classic way to treat such a hysterical fit. We saw this in the old movies, where men hit women because they were hysterical... Shocked, the girl stopped screaming instantly, then cried a bit and calmed down. M, absolutely fearful by now, having hit a patient, saw herself dismissed on the spot. She thought the patient would report her. She did not, and apparently they got on very well afterwards.

Patients used to go in and out of the ward all day, for walks, to the shop, to OT, etc. They came back for their meals and in the evenings. One of them would regularly go for a walk on visitors' day, well dressed, clean, rosy face and bright eyed, and come back about two hours later absolutely filthy, with torn clothes, and stinking, but with a smile on her face. She had got cigarettes...in exchange for her favours... Though we were responsible for her she was a free agent, we could not stop her, but she was put on the pill, as soon as it came on the market.

Years and years later I met a man whose wife had been a patient in Hellingly for several months, suffering from severe puerperal depression, in the seventies. He mentioned casually that he used to take his wife to the woods to "make love" to her on visiting days...opinions are divided on the subject. I felt sorry for the woman, who would not be able to have a choice in the matter, in her condition. I may be wrong...

Arlington and Bodiam were training wards, caring for the "sick and the infirm", mostly the elderly, some with severe learning and physical disabilities, senility of one kind or another, some unable to walk, talk, feed themselves, or even eat ordinary food. These were often called the "babies". One did not have a

41

stomach, she had to be fed liquid food; but she used to pick her blanket and swallow the threads. Anyone who was nursing then will remember the outcome. It was not very nice to deal with! Occasionally younger women with their full thinking capacities had to be nursed in either of these two wards, if they needed intensive care. We felt rather sorry for them as it must have been very depressing to be surrounded by all these very infirm old people, in the worst stages of their lives.

All these people needed full nursing care. Student nurses stayed in the dormitory with the very sick patients, bed ridden.

There were great characters among the patients nevertheless. Grace was very tall and gangly, walking with the aid of a Zimmer frame, her face made up with lipstick and rouge, and wearing bright jewellery. At night she used to sing some of the old songs at the top of her rather shrill voice. I was torn between amusement and dismay as I did not want the other patients to wake up. She was of a cheerful disposition and had a terrific will. She was in charge. When she had a prolapse Dr Gosling fitted her with a pessary. Well, within an hour there she was walking around, grandly, with the pessary around her wrist as a bangle! Dr Gosling, another strong character, had another two or three attempts at fitting this pessary, but then even she had to give up.

Another patient, paraplegic, liked to spend her time in the verandah in the summer; she was brown as a berry. She was a bit bossy with us young ones, I found her a bit scary as her language was rough, but she enjoyed a laugh and a gossip with the older staff.

Sr MacDonald had been one of the sisters in Bodiam ward for years. She was probably in her late fifties when I met her. She was not very tall, but large, calm and quiet. She seemed to walk with difficulty, as in pain, maybe because of her weight, or arthritis, but she never moaned. I found her warm and caring.

When I was on night duty I liked the way how she arrived every morning half-hour early to go by each bed, lift the bedclothes so she could see the patient's faces, and greeted everyone: "Good-morning" by their names.

She delegated most of the clinical duties to the Staff-Nurse but took care of the laundry, some other unpleasant jobs and most of the paperwork as well, assisting and discussing patients with the doctor who was there most mornings. She was in her office a great deal of the time but did not miss anything. She was quite astute, a good judge of people, and would quietly interfere if she felt something was amiss. I got to know her better as a third year student, then as a staff nurse, and when she became ill. She was nursed in the infirmary, where it was my privilege to look after her, during my shifts on Bodiam.

The other sister was an energetic, no nonsense woman, and straightforward; you knew exactly where you were with her. (Was her name Sr.Thompson, as I think it was?) I liked her too. She tried to teach me to express myself more clearly than I did. She asked me once whether something had been done, I knew it had been done but replied: "I think so sister!" She corrected me "you think so or you know so, nurse, so what is it?" "I know so sister!" I liked the way she talked, briskly and to the point, using interesting words and expressions like "You can pop off now nurse".

As a first year student I had more to do with the Staff Nurses. I recall Pat Whippy, second in command. She was a bright and very pretty young English woman, modern, chatty, dynamic, positive and sensible. I aspired to be like her. Ruth Gearing, who was German, was also pretty but forceful, the kind of woman who would call a spade a "bloody shovel". She could be very intimidating, a bit of a tartar, but warm and likeable with it. Both Staff Nurses were very knowledgeable and keen to teach us; this was part of their duties anyway.

I was in Bodiam ward when I passed my final exam. I had noticed right from the start that some French auxiliary nurses thought it was great having one of their compatriots in charge because they felt they could take liberties. I decided to have none of that. From the time I became responsible for junior staff I made sure not to be my usual sweet self. Straight and to the point, pleasant but cool, only speaking English. I relaxed a bit after a while when I felt everyone understood the order of things. Once I was with two other French N/As who had been working with me for a while; we were stock taking in the store cupboard and chatting at the same time. One of the girls remarked to me: "When I first met you I thought you'd be a really good sister!"

"Did you?" said I, practically preening,

"Yes, you looked a right cow!"

Well believe it or not, I was pleased! Talk about a double-edged compliment though. .

Besides the usual nursing tasks, on Sunday afternoons, while the visitors were in the dining /sitting room with their relatives, we in the dormitory quietly sat around a table, filling little paper bags with cotton wool balls, gauze swabs, tongue depressors, and probably other things I cannot remember, to be sent for sterilization. As in other wards, we had a large sterilizer in the clinic for the clinical instruments used in various procedures. (medical examinations, dressings, etc) At this point comes to mind the person turning up after someone died, to collect the eyes as the family had given a written permission. I still find this abhorrent …

Laying out bodies is a gruesome task; I am told that now morticians come to the ward to collect the deceased. I don't know how I did it, looking back on it now. We had to. Only once did I want to run away and be sick: I was not prepared; I was in the middle of some mundane task when a nurse called

44

me from behind the curtains to come and give her a hand. My mind on the living, when I came face to face with the body, a person I knew well, it was as though someone punched me in the stomach. However I rallied round and carried on doing what was to be done. It is strange how minds are able to switch off and become focused on what is to be done.

Night duty started at 9pm. In Bodiam ward by that time everyone was in bed having had their cups of milk, Ovaltine, or such like in bed about 7pm. The ward was quiet, most patients would be asleep. I would stay in the sick dormitory, by the fire, sitting in front of a table. The sickest of the patient was in bed on my right usually, so I could observe her constantly. I remember well one very frail confused and very agitated lady who had to have cot sides around the bed to stop her from getting out. She could not walk but she could try and climb over the cot sides with her great thin long legs and it was a job for me to stop her. Miss Lulham, the night Assistant Matron came to my rescue and gave her a prescribed sedative. The round nurses came every two hours, they were there to help you if you needed, and checked the people in the back dormitory for wet beds. (Some of my colleagues remember a nurse in the back dormitory but I am pretty sure it was not so in the early sixties). In the sick dormitory all incontinent patients (most were) had to be put on the commode, at least twice a night, around 10pm, then around 2am. This took a good hour if not more. This was a tough job on your own, and let's face it we usually did it on our own, unless a patient was really too heavy. But it had its rewards: I recall this old lady telling me as I took her in my arms to get her on the commode, "Oh mum, I don't want to go to school today!" I told her "All right darling, you don't have to!"

We wrote our night's report on separate sheets for each patient to be sent to the Nursing Office in the morning. Most reports were perfunctory when the night had been quiet, but as I thought it must have been boring for the Assistant Matrons to read the same old thing I often gave a blow by blow account of what had gone on, to vary the menu; for instance Grace's rendition of a song. No one ever commented, or told me off. Note writing is strictly controlled now. In my last year at work one of my colleagues was reprimanded for having written that a patient had made her a cup of tea. She was told it should not have been noted as it was not part of her Care Plan…Is it me?

ARLINGTON ward was a mixture of strict order, discipline and confusion, all the result of Sr.White's personality. She had been a sister there for many years. It was often remarked she knew her stuff and was extremely knowledgeable, and she probably was, but by the time I met her she was also quite scatty. We all remember her for her eccentricities. Her unpredictability made it difficult for us to know what we should be doing at any given point. This alone made her rather formidable.

She lived in Hailsham and changed into her uniform on the ward on arrival. (There were changing rooms, but obviously not for the likes of her) She would do so walking around the ward, checking what was going on, telling us what to do, all this time half dressed, for instance one side of her bib pinned, the other dangling, her hair down, which she put up in an elaborate 1940ish style. Once, when I was a 2nd year student nurse she stopped me doing whatever it was, calling me by one of my colleagues' surname, and asked me if I could take a blood pressure. "Yes sister!" said I. "Good! Go and do the cobwebs in the verandah!" she replied. All the while she was eating her breakfast, a bowl of cereal in one hand, sleeve down one arm without a cuff and the other sleeve rolled up with the cuff on her bare arm.

Everyone has a story to tell about Sr. White and her cats. Most wards had at least one cat, she had several, never less than three. Staff would bring her their sickly moggies and she gave them injections of penicillin from the clinic. Saucers of food and milk were scattered around the ward. One of the cats, very large, had a special bed to sleep on in the veranda. I was interested to read a report in Hellingly Park Trust news recently, that they had at last managed to get rid of the feral cats in the area. You can be sure they were the descendants of Sr. White venerated cats!

Female dormitories always had to be spotless and very tidy. In Arlington ward this was carried to extremes. The corners and the lining up of the beds were of paramount importance to Sr White. When she had nothing better to do, we thought, she would interrupt us doing whatever we were doing and summon us back to the empty dormitory. "Come with me nurse!" She would position herself at the end of the line of beds, already made, and follow the line of her hand with her eye to see if any bed was slightly out. Usually you could not see even an inch of difference, but she did, asking you to correct it; thankfully she walked off before you started on the task, so you could pretend to do it as soon as her back was turned.

She hoarded all kinds of things bought for the patients, items of clothing, sweets, chocolates, toiletries, in a store room. These would occasionally come out when the fancy took her. If she wanted to be nice to you she would graciously and benevolently hand you a chocolate bar. We had to pretend to be grateful even when we knew the chocolate was inedible, grey with age. I never had the privilege to actually walk in that room, it must have been a bit like Aladdin's cave. Leone, a friend and ex-colleague, told me that she was once given the key to this inner sanctum when she was a Staff Nurse. Sister had to trust her with it as she was going on leave. My friend found the place stinking of rotten fruit and dirty clothes. Apparently Sister used to get the staff to dress the patients with their personal clothes on visiting afternoons, to take off immediately after the visitors had left and replace them in the store room, often soiled! The rest of the week they wore unnamed ward dresses (but clean). In this store room Leone also found mountains of brand new night-dresses. She decided to sort the room out (she was brave!) distributed what she could to the patients, made large fruit salads and placed a new nightie in each patient's locker. She realised Sister would not be very happy about it, so on her return she presented her with this "fait accompli" as diplomatically as she could. Sister was quiet, she seemed to approve, she could not say anything, and after all there was nothing wrong with what had been done. It was commendable. However the next day Sister returned all the nighties to the store cupboard... because the patients would need them if they had to go to the General Hospital in an emergency! As if!

Our nursing tasks there were similar to the ones in Bodiam. We had severely ill patients to nurse in the sick dormitory and in a little side room. In the very early sixties there were two patients with Tuberculosis nursed in the verandah for isolation and fresh air. Their beds were surrounded with the screens on wheels we used to have then, before proper screens were installed around each bed. These screens had to be sprayed with water regularly for cross infection barrier. How this was supposed to stop the infection spreading, I still wonder...We wore appropriate protective gear; masks etc. and it must have been the more isolating for these people, away from the rest of the ward.

I did not like Arlington on night duty because of the cockroaches. They came down in droves from the central heating pipes and circulated in the corridors. No doubt all the cat food lying about brought them along. I waged a war on them. I used to spray lakes of insect killer on the floor and brush them all into that, then into a pan at the end of the night, (I am sorry about this, animal lovers!) but every night there were more. I had nightmares about them.

On night duty we had more opportunity to get close to some of the patients as we had more time, and when they were at their most vulnerable possibly. I was fond of this ex Tiller girl, with only one leg, the other had been amputated, I can't remember why. She was a dear old lively and brave cockney woman with plenty to say but very confused about the here and now. Regularly incontinent at night she complained bitterly once about the state of the roof, as her bed was soaked...

A girl of nineteen or so was in Arlington ward for a time. She had thrown herself off a second storey window of the hospital and was very lucky to survive. She sustained several fractures and could not walk, needing full nursing care. This girl was well known in the hospital as extremely difficult. She threw tantrums, attacked staff, threatened and attempted to harm herself in all kinds of ways.

I was on night duty during her stay; over the weeks she changed so much she became a pleasure to be with. The only patient we could converse with, she had us to herself, we could give her attention, have discussions, and we became friends. This girl's mental health improved as well as her physical health, due to the one-to-one she had with professionals, nurses particularly. There was also the human physical contact she had to receive, and the mothering that could have been something she lacked. She could not run away from us after all!

I must not forget to mention the works department's role in the ward life. Should anything be needed or repaired we gave them a call and hey presto! A chap came along with a smile and a small chit for us to fill, a little banter, and sorted the problem out promptly, without all the fuss and all the forms there are now. There was much good will all around. I remember the time when I got an inkling that things were changing: one Sunday, I was in charge of Arlington ward, it was bath time as usual. We had our list prepared. A new male nurse was with me. A middle-aged man, he had just joined us after years working in a factory. The bathroom was ready, towels, night clothes ready on a trolley, bath drawn, the first patient undressed just about to go in, when the light bulb went! Being Sunday the works department was closed. I knew we kept light bulbs for emergencies in the office so off I went to get one, and proceeded to fit it myself. The new chap was astounded! Rightly, I now know, he told me the unions would go up in arms about it, probably start a strike, and we should stop the bathing straightaway. Stuff and nonsense, said I, or words to this effect. I knew what both sisters would have to say if they were told the next day that no one was bathed because of a dud light bulb! It occurs to me now how things have changed. The situation would still not be acceptable today but for a different reason. Not to protect the workers, but to protect the management in case of litigation, if I had hurt myself.

Fairlight ward was a small admission ward. The medical staff there was more memorable than the patients. Dr M. the consultant, was a tall, grey, lined, badly-weathered man in his fifties. He smoked continually. He seemed to be in the office every morning, holding court. He was of the Freudian school of thought as all libidinous psychiatrists are - for libidinous read dirty old men - everything related to sex. He was cynical and blasé about everything. Dr Gosling, the registrar, was young, vivacious and pretty. She was one of the few doctors wearing a white coat. She wore it unfastened, and as she strode through everywhere, her mid-length blond hair and her coat flew open with the air she created, reinforcing the impression of great speed. She was terribly nervous when Dr M. was around; she stammered at the best of times, but even more so then. He loved to shock and he must have been rewarded by her reaction. She would become bright red and look extremely uncomfortable.

Half of the time his innuendoes were lost on me, not only because of my poor English, but because I was still quite innocent. I imagined then that she was in love with him, but later on, as I got wiser and got to know her, I revised my assessment. She dreaded him and his bawdy remarks in front of the rest of the staff.

I do remember listening attentively to a psychotic patient in the throes of explaining one of her delusions. I wanted to understand, and you know I nearly did…until I got frightened, I realised if I did not suspend my belief I could go there too.

Alfriston ward catered for acute and disturbed psychotic patients in the sixties. Sr Peggy Knowles was lovely, young and cheerful; she was chatty and protective of her staff. She surprised me the first time I found her sweeping the floor herself as this needed to be done. You would not have seen many of the other sisters demeaning themselves in that way! Besides being pretty she was very with it, with her hair backcombed and she jived and twisted away with the rest of us at parties. As for her counterpart, Sr W, she was a bit of a dragon. She was very butch, slim, with a worn-out face, her dry white/yellow hair in a French pleat beneath her sister's cap, usually with a cigarette between her lips. Her voice was gruff, and she looked tough. But, as with other sisters of the same ilk, her bark was worse than her bite. Some of my colleagues have good memories of her; I have no bad ones, she did not worry me. I was still in my first year, I would not have dreamt of questioning her authority and got on with the work. However a story goes that sometime in the late forties or early fifties a young student nurse was very upset with her for being callous with a particular patient. Frustrated and helpless, in those days you would not have dared reporting your seniors, this young nurse walked off the ward in a fury; on her way downstairs, unable to contain herself any

51

further, she lashed out and broke one of the stairwell windows! I don't know if it calmed her down but when she went back to the ward two days later she found out that this same patient was to receive ECT because she had had a relapse: she had supposedly broken a window…

In the seventies this ward became the "Token Economy Project" ward. Helen Dalton, recently reminisced about her work in that locked ward after she left the Day Patients in Park House in 1978. Psychologists pioneered this project, a novel approach for behaviour modification.

Many of the patients had long histories of destructive or unsociable behaviour problems; some would have been in Broadmoor had they not been accepted by Alfriston ward; others had Eating or Obsessive-Compulsive-Disorders. Medication was not allowed except for one particular chap. Nurses carried little bags of tokens with different colours to reward good behaviour, and each patient had a different colour. Bad or undesirable behaviour would mean withdrawal of something valued, for instance not being allowed visitors. Patients with violent behaviour were taken to a Time-out room with a nurse in attendance until they calmed down. Anorexic patients were weighed regularly; they gained tokens if they put on weight, (some put ball bearings in their pockets to move the scale in their favour.) These tokens were spent in the shop for Cigarettes or other goodies, all much prized.

No one was allowed on the ward without prior notice. The reason was that occasionally, some women would walk around stark naked just for devilment, or make very lewd remarks to male visitors, trying to get a reaction from them. The policy was to ignore this kind of behaviour completely.

Helen found the work rewarding on the whole but extremely taxing; she even nearly got strangled once! She trained in Social

Skills to run very successful groups. She tells me that through this Token Economy regime five out of twenty patients were discharged well. This is not bad considering most had had intensive treatment before with no improvement.

I worked in Chailey ward during my 2nd year of training. This ward cared for women with severe psychotic disorders. It was a bright ward in its layout, and clean as a new pin; order reigned. Strong personalities, staff and patients, often made this ward tense as hell. Sr. Ford was the one to fear; she was another of these big, tall, solid women who spoke as they found. She was a good teacher. With her I learnt to lay a clinical trolley to perfection. We cleaned it all over with methylated spirit first, then placed all sterilised stainless steel instruments on the top shelf, forceps, scissors, gallipots, bowls, kidney dishes, etc. etc. all in strict order. On the bottom shelf we placed the packs of cotton wool balls, bandages, and what have you. Sister would inspect it meticulously and if she found the trolley not up to her standards we had to try again until perfect. The appearance of the trolley was just as important as it being germ free. It had to shine; as methylated spirit leaves smears it was not that easy. But the end result was always pleasing to the eye as far as I was concerned as well. Sr. Reed, though brisk, straight, outspoken and energetic I found easier to relate to.

I had a hair-raising experience in Chailey, one afternoon. Sr. had gone to tea, I was left with a young auxiliary nurse, so I was in charge! It was a nice peaceful afternoon, most of the patients were in Occupational Therapy in the Hall, only two or three patients to look after and they seemed contented in the sitting room. Even N. was knitting. We had been given the task of breaking all the chipped crockery in the kitchen in order for them to be condemned and replaced. To do so we had to fill a pillowcase with the crockery and, with a small wooden hammer, we had a smashing time. That day, while my colleague was in the kitchen looking for the crockery, I was in the sitting room waiting for her, when suddenly N., a hefty thirty-two year old, but acting as a three year old with Attention Deficit Disorder, as big as a volcano, and as unpredictable, decided to throw her knitting in the fireplace, where a fire was lit (yes!).

Now this knitting was an achievement for N. Her mother particularly was proud of it. I was in a dilemma for a few seconds. My natural reaction was to let her, but I debated how both sisters would react. Sr. Reed would not mind but Sr. Ford would, I thought. So I quickly intervened, taking the knitting from her hands before it was too late, telling her she could not do that. She turned on me then, or rather stood, high above me, glaring and breathing over me, (the sweetish smell of medication in her breath comes back to mind) grabbing me by the tops of my arms. Strangely enough, rather than being frightened I felt angry. I had the wooden hammer in my hand and, worried that I might hit her with it, I threw it away, while calling the nurse in the kitchen, as normally as I could. Talking, we managed to get her to her bed in the dormitory, as per policy, and calm her down; all this without violence which would have been negative and impossible for the two of us in any case. Furthermore we had coped without drugs, inaccessible to us. I stayed with her for a little while, tucking her in, and she was fine. Afterwards we respected each other and I had no more problems with her.

In any ward, or in the community, individually or in groups, some patients have to test staff in charge they do not know, to see how untoward situations will be handled. Most of us need to know the boundaries and to feel safe I suppose.

Sr. Ford surprised me once by showing a mischievous side to her nature. We were both in the dormitory when through the door we caught sight of Miss McC., one of the Assistant Matrons, creeping towards the office door, on her toes, as silently as she could, to catch Sister out no doubt. Sister smiled at me, put her finger across her mouth to make sure I kept quiet and then quickly jumped out, singing with a booming voice: "Tiptoe through the tulips..." This song always brings her to mind with a smile.

It was in this ward one evening that one of my young colleagues and myself were reprimanded by an SEN for having too much fun when brushing the patients' dentures! This made us even more cheerful. In fact we had been talking about this task, amongst others, that we would never have contemplated doing before we came to the hospital, but did as part of the job without thinking.

A similar thing happened in Bodiam ward when I was making beds with another French girl, gossiping about the young men in the club. As young girls do, we were giggling away, when the SEN popped her head in the dormitory to tell us spitefully that she knew we were talking about her! After a moment of surprise we burst into laughter more heartily than before of course! We felt she was annoyed that we were having fun, we also thought she was paranoid. Again, we were young, and as we spoke French, she could not understand us. But we did not think we had to speak English when no one else was around. And why should we?

A few months later, at the end of my second year I was sent to take charge of Danehill, a non-training geriatric ward, one afternoon when the sister was off. This was fine, by then I was confident in running a ward, having practised with supervision from sisters and staff nurses. However the SEN in that ward was one of the old league, let's call her Nurse Bully Boots, as we all knew her to be a terror, particularly with us young ones. She had even slapped a colleague's face once. Again let me say that it was only a handful of untrained old-timers, with chips on their shoulders, resenting us.

She stayed in attendance as I took the hand-over from the Sister on the morning shift. As soon as we were alone she told me she was in charge. No, said I, I knew the ranking order and what I was there for. She was livid; "Well I won't tell you anything about the ward and I won't let you have the keys to the private cupboard, I have them in my pocket!" she replied. "Never mind I shall cope" said I. And I did. Sister had told me the afternoon agenda. Wards were really well organised. You could walk in and have lists of everything to do, and in what order. So that was no problem; besides I had a couple of good nurses with me who knew the ward and the patients. As BB usually harassed them they rallied round me very happily; we were a nice team! I was not worried, but not having the keys to the cupboard on visiting day was a problem, as this held the patients' coats.

I managed nevertheless by explaining to the relatives that the key was missing and would they mind borrowing one of the ward's stock? Nobody did mind, everyone was kind. Meanwhile BB was in the kitchen keeping an eye on the proceedings and discussing the situation over a cup of tea with a porter, glaring at me as I was passing by. She disappeared for more than an hour at tea-time. Believe me I really would have preferred she stayed away altogether. During her extended break she must have had a grand old time moaning about me as I got several phone calls to congratulate me in my dealings with her. "Well done Ruppert!" was the consensus of opinions... It occurs to me now that the Nursing Office might have warded me there to see how I would manage the situation. They were astute women, these assistant matrons, and could be mischievous, and they knew us all. They had been on the wards themselves so they had a good idea of what went on.

Now older I realize it must have been galling to have these young chits of girls, just off the boat, decide what there was to do and who should do it. The funny thing is how these women changed their attitude towards us when we became Staff Nurses. My dealings with BB after this contretemps were… Oh so harmonious! Just sweetness and smiles.

Amberstone, built in the 1950s, a new addition to Hellingly hospital for acute neurosis admissions, was modern and bright and spacious. It was a world apart, where patients and staff felt privileged to be. We were not supposed to, but sometimes nurses would try and manipulate patients to cooperate by threatening them with the main building. Amberstone was often thought to be for the elite, but I don't really think so. Patients had the same staff looking after them and received similar treatments, though the building was modern. Rumour had it that in the past a psychiatrist's wife was treated there for depression under the name of Mrs X, after a broken love affair.... Allegedly her own husband had prescribed ECT...

Upstairs, a long corridor separated the male and female sides. There were many single rooms with a large dormitory for the new admissions at each end of the building. There was a clinic, a 6 bedded room, also used for insulin or ECT treatments, a mother and baby unit started in 1968/69, bathrooms and a little kitchen for staff and patients beverages.

Downstairs male and female, patients and staff, shared the facilities: a communal living room/sitting room, a state of the art large hall for social and recreational activities, and a dining room. Patients could choose their favourite meal from the varied menus prepared by the chef on the premises, in a large kitchen. This integration of the sexes made for an altogether more normal and relaxed atmosphere different from working in the main building.

Many patients were very young, and in my first spell there, as a junior nurse of twenty, I enjoyed the company of two girls around my age. Looking back I cannot think what could have been the matter with them! One may have been a bit anxious, she may have had panic attacks, but the other one was cheerful, bright as a penny, and lively. We had great fun together. We were further united in our dread of Sister B. She was rather unusual looking at that time, in her uniform; she wore the Sister's cap over her long red hair in large ringlets falling well below the collar, and a lot of make up. Flouting all the rules she got away with it. Very colourful, she was forceful and had a temper. I got to know her better some ten years later in Park House, she had not changed but I had; she did not frighten me any longer. I liked her spirit, she could be great fun..

One of the patients in Amberstone, a lady in her forties, suffered with anorexia as a reaction to her husband leaving her for another woman. When she came to us she was so frail she could hardly walk. I have this picture in mind of both of us in the mirror, my chubby self preferring my body and mind to hers; she like a skeleton with the skin on, but unable to see the state she was in. Due to her illness she had lost her hair and wore voluminous glamorous wigs which made her look horrific. I liked her, she was a sweetie; she was also very bright and well read. With a laugh she called me "La Belle Dame Sans Merci" as I would stay with her until she managed to accomplish whatever she had to do on her own.

My first night in Amberstone was in 1964. The Sister, another of those formidable big women, took me up to the little room next to the ladies's dormitory and introduced me to the male nurse, telling him to show me the ropes. She then made her way back to her office, situated downstairs by the main entrance.

This young man told me how to make myself comfortable, with two chairs, a pillow and a blanket. He also took me through a short relaxation session so I could be cosy and drop off to sleep… No way could I sleep, I was too nervous, I could not even relax.

As for him he soon dropped off while I read. About an hour or so later sister came up the stairs, very noisily, coughing her lungs out. (She was a chain smoker and died of lung cancer a few years later). Thinking that it was perfectly all right for the young chap to sleep, I did not wake him up. Sister read him the riot act… I was so ashamed and contrite that I apologised to him as soon as Sister went out, feeling very silly not to have guessed we were not allowed to sleep; however he did not seem to be fazed and remained pleasant to me. As young and naïve then, I found the male staff usually very educative regarding their view on women. For instance, according to most, all girls who rejected them were gay. Once I was told by a rather drippy boy that the depressed women in the ward needed a real man to cure them. Annoyed, I told him that in that case it was unfortunate for them as there was none around but him…

Reading has always been a must for me and I was desperate for a book after a month in England. I soon discovered Agatha Christie in the hospital library. She was the author for me: easy to read and enjoyable, her books written in clear and perfect English, the plots made for riveting reads. By the time I was on night duty in Amberstone I was ready for something more substantial. Assisted by a French/English dictionary I got into the life of Elizabeth I, a very thick and scholarly tome. It took me a while, though I have to admit I skipped most of the war passages as I found them too tedious, but after this hard work I could get into practically anything.

During the break we cooked our meals in the vast main kitchen downstairs, using the giant stainless steel fryers used during the day for about fifty people. Being there felt a bit spooky, every noise echoed in that room.

Prize
Giving
1967

Back row   Eddie Longhorn - ? -John Parson - Paul Organ - Stuart McMullan - Nevil Smith - Norman Turton
Middle row   Bridget Freaks - Nicole Parmainteny - Celia Sullivan - Charlyne Bidois - Nino - Sylvia Trusler - ? - Christine Mansman - me -
                Mrs Leak - Jeannine Turton
Front row   John Foord - Mr G. Gutteridge - Senior Nurse GNC, Chairman of the Management Committe - Miss Bradley, Matron -
                and Dr Rice, Medical Superintendent

60

Nurses' Prize Giving
2nd November 1967

Awards

GOLD MEDAL: Honours Certificate: Mrs. R. Waterson

SILVER MEDAL: Honours Certificate: Mr. M.A. Elliott

BRONZE MEDAL: Honours Certificate: Mr. J.B. Foord

HONOURS CERTIFICATE AND HOSPITAL BADGE: Miss R.V. Field

HOSPITAL BADGES AND CERTIFICATES

Mr. N. Waterson	Mrs.M. Tagoe	Mrs. E.M.Leake
Mrs. J. Turton	Mr. J. Parsons	Miss E.J. Ruppert
Mr. N. Smith	Mr. R.J. Clark	Miss C.A. Mansmann
Mr. N. Turton	Miss S.H. Trusler	Mr. S. Preziusi
Mr. J.L. Carraz	Mr. J.M. Stepney	

INTERMEDIATE EXAMINATION PRIZES

OCTOBER 1966	Miss C. Sullivan	Mr. S.V. McMullan
JUNE 1967	Mr. P.I. Organ	Mrs. N. Parmainteny

SUBJECT PRIZES

JUNIOR PSYCHIATRY:	Mr. J.F.C. Kennard	Miss C. Ronzani	Miss C.H.E. Bidois
SENIOR PSYCHIATRY:	Mrs. E.M. Leake	Mrs. H.B. Cassidy	Miss B. Freakes
PSYCHO-PHYSICAL DISORDERS:		Mrs. R. Waterson	Miss R.V.Field
		Mr. M.A.Elliott	
PRACTICAL & ORAL PRIZE:		Mr. J.B. Foord	

TUTOR'S PRIZES

Mrs. N. Parmainteny   Mr. P.I. Organ

PRINCIPAL NURSING OFFICER'S PRIZES

Mrs. E.M. Leake   Mr. S. Preziusi

In the main hospital male and female staff integrated gradually from 1967, in ranking order. I was the first Staff Nurse to work on a male ward, GUESTLING. This was a culture shock to say the least!

Women were not welcome in this male dominated world; it was very lackadaisical as far as order and cleanliness were concerned. There were other practices in G1, well against everything we had learnt and stood for. The Charge Nurse, an old timer, was pally with the male nursing officers. He really upset me once, as he shouted at a poor old man I was talking to because he had sweet papers in his pockets; he then gave him a clip on the head before telling him to go away. May-be he thought his bullying tactics would impress me. When he walked out of the room I was very irate. A few minutes later he showed his face just for a minute, just enough to let me know he had heard me in the middle of sounding off to one of my male colleagues about what I had seen. I had said that I could not bear to work in those conditions, which were going against all the principles we had been taught, that I had a good mind to report him, and on and on... (I could see the student nurse thought I was over the top and was trying to calm me down, and that did not help). I was a bit shocked that the brute had heard me but also pleased he knew my reaction to his behaviour. I did not witness any more bullying... He left not long after, eloping with the Sister on the opposite shift, a married woman who was one of the first Sisters given a ward on the male side (so much for integration). You may remember my mention of this event, of this couple who went with most of the content of the store cupboard...

I came back to Guestling, on part-time day duty in May 1972. The hospital had undergone massive changes in two years. Miss Bradley had retired and died in quick succession, she was replaced by Miss Crichton who I never met, as she left a few months after my return. Mr Reinhold succeeded her.

Besides the male and female staff being fully integrated, the patients had also all been moved to different wards according to their residential areas. This must have been a major upheaval for several months for everyone throughout the whole hospital. By then I had two young children to bring up on my own and I felt very lucky to be able to work at all; I could use the hospital crèche, another innovation. Its hours were from 9am to 5pm, for children below school age; this was great. I was doubly fortunate, as shortly before I applied to come back, for about a year, part-time work had not been allowed. This rule had only recently been rescinded. However to start with, my working hours, to coincide with the crèche's, caused me some friction with one or two staff. They threw barely veiled remarks that there was nothing for me to do by the time I arrived on the ward at 9am. I even got the impression that they rushed to get the patients up, dressed and breakfasted in order to show me I was useless. Anyway there was plenty for me to do, besides making all the beds on my own on arrival, and I soon felt accepted as a useful member of the team.

Guestling was now for the female "sick and elderly" patients, in Hastings and Rother area. I remember Mr Bradley was one of the Charge Nurses. He was pleasant, kind and easy going, a great difference from the previous C/N I had worked with four years earlier. Another important change was that most staff, other than Sisters and Charge Nurses, now addressed each other by their first names rather than surnames. This added to the casual atmosphere as a rule.

One particular patient in Guestling was for me an example of how you could ruin your life. She had attempted to take hers by overdosing with Aspirin. From being depressed and able bodied, she became totally paralysed and had come to an elderly ward in a psychiatric hospital for full nursing care, treatment of her depression and physical rehabilitation. This was a really terrible turn of event for her who had wanted to be free of whatever she thought was wrong with her life. Our task was to re-educate her into dressing, walking and feeding herself, as well as helping her to accept her lot, if not to be happier in herself. She needed much encouragement. She learnt to walk with callipers and with a leather contraption around her wrist she could hold a spoon in her hand and feed herself unaided. Eventually she became well enough to be transferred to a residential nursing home several months later. To me then, her life had all the elements of tragedy. But now I wonder whether I was judging the situation subjectively, because of my own independent personality. She may have found her invalidity meant she had support, contact and company, which she may have craved for previously, when she lived on her own and took the overdose. Who knows? But to me her's has always been a cautionary tale.

I worked in Jevington ward around the same period. I often made the sandwiches in the kitchen for the patients' tea, assisted by a patient from Amberstone. She told me the cause of her depression. It occurs to me this was my first "counselling" session as such. I had recovered from a similar experience to her's and we both found talking together helped. It was also good to know that I had gained understanding from my ordeals.

Another patient from Park House came to play the piano for the old folks for a while. Once I found this lady playing away with all the patients in their armchairs, locked in the sitting room with her! When I asked the staff why the door was locked, I was told the ambulant ladies could not bear this music/noise and they would walk out otherwise! They did not want the pianist upset! I had to laugh.

Until then I had been used to Sisters and Charge Nurses having the final word. The first time I saw this rule crumble was very soon after a young male nursing assistant joined us: we had had our elevenses with Sr. Vine, and after the usual few minutes we got up to resume our duties. Well, not all of us: the young man sat still, reading his paper…Sister noticed it so she told him to get off his backside and join us. He replied he would when he was good and ready! We were all flabbergasted! Yes, integration was the beginning of the end for the NHS! I am not sure I am joking…

Park House is special to me. The first ward I had walked into on my arrival at the hospital, I was warded there time and again; on day and night duty, as a Student Nurse, Staff Nurse and eventually in charge of the Day-Patients department from 1974. Finally I left Hellingly from Park House, with the Day-Patients department, in 1982 - and on the personal side, my boy-friend's room was on the left of Park House entrance in the early sixties…it became the Nursing Officer's Secretary's office…

I cannot pass by Park House nowadays without a pang of nostalgia to see it so abandoned. There used to be an old fashioned bench made of logs on the roadside by the drive in front of Park House. It was very picturesque even if not very comfortable to sit on; in the seventies a common or garden looking one replaced it.

Originally there was Park House East and Park House West. I was interested to hear that Canadian Soldiers were billeted there during WWII when one of these soldiers presented himself at our office one day to ask if he could visit the building. He was very moved and wistful, recalling his good memories about the place.

I worked with various staff at different times. I cannot remember all their names, though I have very good vibes about several. On day duty Sr. Ross was the first sister I worked with in Park House. She was bright, energetic, quick and efficient; she did not suffer fools gladly. She made me a little bit nervous. But at the time nobody terrified me as much as Dr Gosling. Now she did not suffer fools at all, and most were fools as far as she was concerned! A bundle of nerves and very mercurial she flew off the handle for the smallest of things and shouted at whoever was in the way. You may remember my mentioning her stammer before, but when she was really rattled, and this was often, her words could not come out. One morning, when I was in the dormitory with the patients, she charged in asking for Sister. I could not help her. So, as red in the face as were her stockings, incandescent with anger, she spluttered and stuttered at me. She had lost me. I was paralysed, a mouse in front of a wild cat. All I could think was that I could not understand a word she said; her hysteria had communicated itself to me. This did not help either of us. It was clear she thought me a waste of space, I understood that very clearly; and so she stormed out to find someone else. I tried to keep out of her way for a long time after that.

Her notes fascinated me; she had strong reactionary opinions (that is the kindest way I can put it) on everything. In her very clear, pale blue, easy to read copperplate writing, she wrote quirky judgmental medical reports on the patients which, I am ashamed to admit, were fun reading. Every sentence brought some sarcastic comment like: "She walked in the office like a duck in a thunderstorm", "Looking as though she was sucking a lemon" or "A ship in full sail". I know these now as hackneyed sentences, clichés, but to me then they were novel. She wrote to entertain. We were taught in school to keep to facts and not be critical, but she obviously did not care. Others above her could be equally judgmental in their note writing. It said more about them than about the patients…

Later, when I was in charge of Amberstone on night duty, in 1969, Dr Gosling who lived in the building often came to my office late at night along with her cats; as we chatted she brushed them while they walked on my desk, their fur flying all over the place! I did not mind, I was amused, she was good company by then, I was no longer terrified of her. Though I could not agree with some of her beliefs, by then we had got to know and respect each other.

New admissions in Park House, as in any other ward, were seen as soon as possible after their arrival by the ward doctor who gave them a full medical, mental and neurological examination; tests were requested from the Path Lab for analysis. For their first three days patients stayed in their night attire, in bed or sitting down in the dormitory for observation. At least one nurse had to be in situ in the dormitory at all times, or else! Patients were escorted to the toilets, washrooms, or bathrooms and we brought their meals on a tray. In the summer they usually sat in the veranda, part of the observation dormitory; it was very pleasant there with the attractive scenery of the woods behind the lawn, with the birds hopping and squirrels running about, picking the leftovers from breakfast!

Then usually over the next few days the patients were allowed to dress and get into the ward routine. No one was allowed to stay on their beds unless they were unwell. Initially they went to Occupational Therapy on the first floor where they were assessed for their preference. There were umpteen possibilities besides the activities in the OT proper, as I noted earlier. Everyone had to be occupied with something or other; nurses in attendance in the dormitory "engaged" and generally "socialised" with the patients; playing scrabble was a great favourite. (One of my friends introduced me at parties thus: "This is Elisabeth, she plays scrabble for a living!"). We took the patients for short walks in the area and the ones not considered at risk went out on their own anywhere as long as they reported their comings and goings to the staff.

The senior staff used to work out a rota for light household duties. (Yes, isn't it dreadful, patients contributing to the daily household chores!). There were always patients vying for kitchen duty (making teas etc.) Women liked to be in charge in the kitchen! I bet they did not have that problem on the male side!

We can all occasionally be judgmental in our approach to the patients. To be fair, when a patient has been acting out, when you are all frazzled at the end of the day, anyone working with the public will believe me, it is difficult to remain with an "unconditional positive regard". To be able to see a situation neutrally most people need time to cool off. Even with your beloved kith and kin it is hard sometimes to remain neutral.

I got my face slapped once, following Sr Hamilton's request to get a patient to get up and have her breakfast in the dining room. I was relaying the message to this lady with an attitude and " slap!" went her hand on my cheek while she said that she was not going to be told what to do by a "chit of a girl!" I was stunned and suddenly became aware of my hand coming up to strike back! Help! I must not, thought I… and with real effort I managed to get my arm back by my side, but I was infuriated… Fired up, I went back to Sister and said: "Sister, she slapped me!" "Did she now, right!" and went to read her the riot act. She would not tolerate any of her staff being hit she told her. I was really pleased to be vindicated but also of having been able to stop myself from retaliating.

One or two years later as a staff nurse I worked with Monique Novak, one of the sisters in Park House then, working opposite

Sr Hamilton. We complemented each other well, and had a similar sense of humour. One morning we were laughing about something or other in the office when a Nursing Officer, always a sombre looking gentleman, walked in on his round. For some reason we became hysterical when he walked in; he may have looked too serious and intense, but anyway we could not stop, he could not get any sense out of us and walked out, back to his office in the main building. We calmed down soon afterwards; one did not fool about with Nursing Officers. Ten minutes later the phone rang: Nanette Carr who had heard of our behaviour from her colleague wanted to know what we had been up to; she said to Monique she had explained our laughter by telling him that she had telephoned us prior to his arrival to warn us his flies were undone! (This was not true by the way!). We did not see him for a while after that...

On night duty at Park House in my early days there was an elderly sister in charge. She stayed in the office all night while I stayed in the dormitory. My experience of this sister is that she slept the nights through. This was particularly annoying one night; a patient who could not sleep asked me for medication around one o'clock in the morning. As sedatives were not given after 2am, for obvious reasons, I had to try and wake sister up, but I just could not, short of shaking her violently; this I did not have it in me to do. She was very frail, not long before her retirement, and might have been deaf as well. At the end of our night she never asked me how it had gone on, as anyone else would have. As for me, I did not have the courage to let her know that one of our patients needed medication to sleep and that I had not been able to wake her, the Sister in Charge, as she had been sleeping so soundly herself. What a shy little thing I was in those days! Anyway I noticed later on that she had written in her report everyone had slept well! Regardless, this experience was positive for both the patient and I learnt to cope without drugs. I also learnt I could use persuasion to get the patient to accept she could do without sedatives. I have to admit I lied to that lady, telling her that Sister did not approve with her having a sedative then. She took it well and did go back to sleep after a cup of tea.

When all were asleep, I would sit in the armchair in the dormitory, wrapped in my cape for warmth, beside the angle poised lamp, reading, while the mice would be scurrying around my feet; (the ward cat was useless, he was too well fed during the day) this was marginally better than the cockroaches in Arlington! I must not forget the constant clanging and banging of the ancient central heating pipes throughout the night...The central heating system in Park House was constantly under repair until finally, about three years or so before it was forever closed, about a million and a half pounds was spent on a new system...

Later on, when I was qualified, confident and in charge at night in Park House East, in the office myself, I found it good to have company, staff or patient who could not sleep. We often had deep and meaningful discussions; we shared more, less on our guard in the small hours.

I did my rounds at 10pm and 2am to check on the patients upstairs. Now one night when I got up the stairs and switched the lights on, something odd occurred. There were two switches for four lights, two came on at a time, but that night, lo and behold, they came in one by one as I advanced through the corridor. This was weird!

There were many ghost stories as usual as in any hospital. A grey lady in Park House, a white lady in Arlington, or it could be the other way around; I did not pay much heed to that. When some people are tired and all is quiet, on the point of dropping off, or waking up, they can have hypnogenic hallucinations; these are

70

nothing to worry about. A friend was convinced she was going psychotic as one night, in one of those drowsy spells; she saw just a big black pair of men's shoes before her eyes, nothing above. I thought it could have been one of the nurses on their rounds not wanting to wake her; we all wore men's shoes!

Some staff reported hearing people running about upstairs occasionally, but when they went upstairs all was quiet, everyone was asleep. Well, this was no mystery to me. Sometimes men crept from the male side to visit our women. I nearly caught what sounded like a little party once. I could hear laughing and shuffling as I was going upstairs. I made sure they knew I was coming by making myself heard, so they could disappear before I arrived on the scene.

Park House East, the female side, was divided into two female admission wards in the early seventies: Camber downstairs and Iden upstairs. George Bordoli, Ruth Gearing, Pat Hackett, Stephen House and Jean Pierre Parmainteny were some of the nurses in charge whose names I recall. Stephen worked in other wards in Park-House from 1976 to 1982 when he went to join the Community Psychiatric Nurses in the Community. He was a very progressive young man and a university graduate to boot. He was very attractive with his long blond hair, blue eyes and engaging smile, and very popular. He had a way about him: as a reluctant (he tells me) branch secretary for COHSE, he managed to get me to stand on the picket line at the bottom of the drive, one lunch-time, during the work-to-rule strike. I would not have done it for anyone else. For my pains some bumptious and well-heeled official in his very expensive car, nearly ran over my foot when all I was doing was trying to give him a leaflet!

At this point let me say the management of the time encouraged us to join one of the Unions when we started work, for our protection. It seems that some staff now feel this is not a useful or necessary thing to do.

Park House West, originally the male side, also turned into two wards: Westfield downstairs was an acute admission ward for men, where Betty Bowman was sister on one of the shifts. We had met in Amberstone years before. Now on a different footing; we got to know each other better. She ran one of the first groups in our area, an encounter group for men with personality problems. She was well equal to it. Upstairs, Dear Gladys Jones was in charge of Beckley, a female rehabilitation ward, preparing patients for discharge. Mary Jo was the Staff Nurse there when I met her. S.he told me recently of a patient who, recovered from a severe illness, was ready for discharge. MB, her Social Worker, came to take her home. Just as they were about to set off, this lady announced that the previous night a naked man had hidden under her bed. Mary Jo could see MB's mind clicking away. Far from being pragmatic, he was well known to have psychoanalytical leanings, and it was a good bet he was analysing the deep Freudian meaning of this event while probably also wondering if she was fit for discharge after all. Mary Jo let him cogitate for a bit, and then she told him: indeed, the night before, one of the new admissions in Westfield had got out of his bed and, naked, had wandered upstairs to hide under the lady's bed! Yes, she was absolutely ready for discharge!

I must not forget the patients' garish rehabilitation flat, made up in the seventies in the middle of Park House, behind the kitchen serving all the wards. To keep up with the trends of the time, each of this flat's walls were painted with different shocking colours in each room. Orange, acid green, purple, etc.; all very psychedelic! This could not have been very restful.

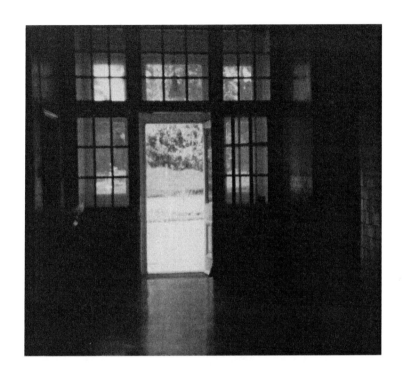

Park House main entrance.... notice the shiny floor!

SOCIAL LIFE AS A LIVING-IN NURSE.

England was the place for the young to be in the sixties. The new pop culture was buzzing, not that we were in the hub of it at Hellingly, but we were close. There was the television I had not had at home, bringing the latest innovations, crazes, Top of the Pops, there were the parties, the cinema, discos; all made you feel alive and I felt the world was right there for me. I never thought it was that permissive though.

If we were not up to walking, brakes provided transport to Hailsham bringing bring the staff to and from work. We picked it up in the High street at the bus stop, by the vicarage field. It was still a field then... There was a rickety barbed-wire fence separating us on the pavement from the cows grazing peacefully in the meadow, with the superb view over the undulating countryside. The hospital water-tower standing imposingly in the horizon made it all the more picturesque. It was there one day, as I waited, watching and listening to children chatting, that I marvelled at their proficiency in the English language!

After the Railway Station closed in 1965 we had to rely on buses to get to Eastbourne or hitch-hike back to the hospital if we did not want to miss the last ten minutes of a film at the cinema in Eastbourne. There were always two features presented in those days. You did not usually know what the first minor film would be; it was often more enjoyable than the main one. I was very keen on all the Agatha Christie's murder mystery films with Margaret Rutherford as Miss Marple; it was all so very English, the settings, the characters, and the music that complemented it so well. Also does anybody remember the silent film, that classic, "The plank", a satire on the construction of new housing estates?

Many of us also went to the "discos" on Saturday nights, (the Cabana and the Catacombs are two names coming to mind). Around midnight all of us girls would be scattered along the road competing for a lift…

During short holiday breaks, usually in pairs, many of us hitch-hiked around Britain. Two of our friends came back from a trip once and were thrilled to report Prince Charles had stopped his Land Rover to give them a lift when he found them walking in the grounds of Balmoral, which was out of bounds; nevertheless he was very charming! They had an enjoyable chat in French and could not wait to tell us.

Some of us hitch-hiked home to the continent for our holidays as well; we had little money, and did what we could. In those days most people were trusting and unafraid. Only once in France did we, my sister and I, come upon a "flasher". I told him psychiatrists could solve that kind of problem and demanded he stopped the car, which he did. He was harmless but the situation was nerve racking all the same.

That first English summer of mine, 1964, was a lovely one, as indeed all the summers seem to have been for me in the sixties… Besides walking I cycled a lot everywhere; it blew the cobwebs and chased the spiders away after work. We were able to borrow bikes from a little shed near the centre, practically any time of the day. I was that keen, I cycled a couple of times in the night to Pevensey after leaving work at 9pm. It took me one hour and a half there and back. (What stamina I had then…) But it was usually in the mornings, after a night at work, that I would pedal my way through the little lanes on the marshes leading to Pevensey Bay, for a swim and a read and a snooze. This was heaven! One such day I had a fantastic experience while cycling in the morning sunshine; the air was pure and balmy, the large sky cloudless in the vast expanse of the marshes; sheep and horses grazing everywhere, tall grasses swaying in the wind as I was coasting along the river, being alone in this landscape; all this contributing to make me feel really free, good and happy. I started singing at the top of my voice and suddenly I became aware of a full orchestra accompanying me! Divine, I tell you, but not something you like to brag about when you work in a mental hospital. This never recurred. Maybe I should get on a bike again... The fact I had not slept and my stomach was empty was no doubt a contributory factor to this experience.

Saving £5 a month out of my £18, I was eventually able to get myself a pair of contact lenses for £50. We could not get them locally then, few people in my walk of life wore them, so I had to go to London, somewhere in Knightsbridge I think, anyway somewhere very swish, every month, for quite a while. Being fitted to requirements was a bit of a palaver but I enjoyed these outings very much. I took the coach from North St, in Hailsham, it always stopped for a cup of tea half-way- I thought it was so quaint- and once in London I walked to my appointment using different routes every time to discover new sites.

Some staff hardly went out of the grounds. It was difficult for many to leave when they retired as they had spent their entire adult life in this community. It was their home. It is a cliché to say it was as easy for the staff to be institutionalised as for the patients. Most people need a supportive environment which the hospital provided. There was also the fact that from time immemorial female nurses had not been allowed to pursue their career if they married. So Matron, most of the assistant matrons, and the older sisters were still single and had had very little life outside. No wonder having to leave was traumatic. Many died shortly after retirement. Of course there were quite a few discreet relationships, of the heterosexual or homosexual kind. (They were not "gay" then.) Everyone knew everybody else's business, gossip was rife and it was hard to keep a secret! I got the definite impression at different times that the biggest crime was to be discovered, or to come clean. For instance I was told from a good witness that a girl who had applied for a job did not get it because she had confessed to having a child out of wedlock; the babe was looked after by his grand-mother and there was no question of him coming to England. I was shocked that the girl's honesty cost her her livelihood.

I also have it on excellent authority that some couples did marry on the quiet and carried on living in their separate nurses' homes until the policy changed. These couples had to creep in and out of each other's rooms. That must have added to the romance!

Of course this kind of thing also happened outside of marriage... How could I forget that evening I came out of my room on the second floor to find J's boy-friend hanging outside on the window ledge, begging to be let in and then to knock on J's door? They had had a row and he did not think she would see him. She did. I thought it great fun and admired his ardour.

I am sure I am not alone in remembering the young couple very primly standing together, side by side, in the corridor, next to the laundry room, every evening, talking earnestly for hours at a time. They did not belong to the so-called permissive society by all appearance. They are married with a family now.

Living and working at the hospital felt safe to me. I found it a good transition from family life and complete independence. As far as I was concerned, the parenting, in the form of Matron and most of her assistants, was benevolent and fair. We would be told off if we did not toe the line but were supported none the less. The organisation with its discipline was more predictable than at home, when one could be subject to the vagaries of parents' moods and fancies.

In the first few months I seemed to be on a constant high. I found it all absolutely wonderful. It felt great to think I could stay up all night, even if I never chose to do so. At home, before I came to England, I had to switch the light off at nine pm, believe it or not. I felt free, proud of earning my own money.

It seemed the natural thing to socialise and form relationships with the local youth at the hospital club. On the other hand, not fluent in the language it could be difficult to sort the wheat from the chaff. I was quiet and reserved then, easily captivated by cheerful banter and attention. I suppose anyone voluntarily leaving the humdrum of family life for another country is not usually attracted to the conventional. Months too late, a sensible young French woman warned me that if I wanted exclusivity I should not pick a boy-friend amongst the staff... I had fallen for a good looking and cheeky blue eyed Irishman with dark hair. He was, with the soft lilt of his accent, master of the blarney. I met him at a party I had not wanted to go to, a month after I arrived at the hospital. I was in the dining room, with two friends who were also newcomers, when a young man approached Mado, the prettiest of us, to ask if she would meet him that night. When she told him she would not go without us he disappeared for a while and came back all excited with the news he had found two other men and so we could have a party... Mado and Annie were keen but I was not. We had quite an argument about it in the nurses' home, but eventually I gave in, they would never have forgiven me. This "party" took place in one of the boys' room, in the male block, where we were forbidden to go... The lights were low, probably provided by candles stuck in a bottle as it was fashionable then, the music was lively to start with; we twisted to the Beatles' hits, "She loves you ye ye ye", and "I want to hold your hand", just out that year. And then the slows started, P asked me to dance to Nat King Cole's "Mary's child" and I was in love. My friends did not click with anyone funnily enough, after all the nagging they had put me through. P and I courted on and off for about two years (we had different aims and objectives, lets put it that way!) then he left for Birmingham... to get married... according to the rumours he may have spread himself...

I moved to The Beeches, a villa back from the drive, around 1966 or 67 after my sister joined me from France. These rooms were prized; there could not have been more than five or six, away from the throng, in the woods. The crème de la crème!

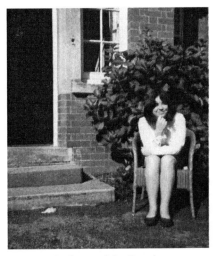

In front of the Beeches
Summer '67

I met my husband to be at another party I did not want to go to, in late 1966. This party was held in the common room. I felt a bit listless, not sociable at the time and intended to stay in my room with a good book. At the last moment I was asked to bring my record player. It seems strange now that mine was the only available one; it came in a neat leather case and you could put several singles on at a time. As I wanted to keep my eye on it I thought I better come to this party after all.

In those days parties always began with boys propping up the bar and girls lined up on chairs against the wall, like the proverbial wallflowers, waiting to be asked for a dance; few girls asked boys. However as soon as some lively music started we girls jumped up to twist and jive and rock in a group until the lads gathered the courage to join us…

Very soon after I moved out of the hospital to a little attic room next to my friend Charlyne, at White Briers, Leap Cross. This house was pulled down very soon after I left it. (It was nothing to do with me, the council wanted to widen London road!)
Chris and I got engaged at my parents' in France in the autumn of 1967. I had qualified as a Mental Nurse in February; we were expected to work the year to repay our training so I fulfilled my obligations with the NHS before leaving in March 1968 to get married and move to Hastings.

TREATMENTS AND THERAPIES

In the sixties Largactil was the drug of choice as a major tranquilliser for people with schizophrenia. It came usually in a liquid form then, easier to administer and less likely for the patients to keep under the tongue or store; however the old ladies occasionally would spit out the sticky stuff in your face…

Long ago the only recourse for disturbed and violent patients who were a danger to themselves or others had been to seclude them. Then Paraldehyde was used extensively for a number of years. This drug had to be administered by intramuscular injection with a large old-fashioned glass syringe as the substance dissolved the plastic ones… This just shows you…And yet, I was reminded recently that many patients had a liking or were even addicted to it. You would know just by walking in a ward if it had been given, by the sickly overpowering smell.

I must have been one of the last nurses to help a patient go through Modified Insulin Therapy. This was given in Amberstone to people with severe depression, in a small dormitory with the curtains closed. There were never more than one or two patients in my experience. They fasted overnight and at 9 am the doctor came to administer the insulin. For the next 2 or 3 hours the nurse attending sat by and observed, took and recorded the patient's temperature, pulse, respiration and blood pressure every half-hour. The patients were in a deep sleep, a mini coma, and perspired freely so we would wipe their brows and make sure they were as comfortable as possible. We woke them up at midday, with a large glass of glucose, then a meal. This treatment was repeated a few times on a weekly basis. It was very effective in treating depression. Patients invariably regained their appetite for food and for living, put on weight and recovered. Was it the sleep, the insulin, or was it the full nursing care they received? Maybe it was a combination of all these factors. This treatment was also discontinued in the seventies, as old fashioned I expect. It demanded at least one nurse for one to three patients in a whole morning. Probably too costly!

I have not assisted at an ECT since the early eighties but I shall try to explain how it had changed over the years. Horrendous stories abound from the past, many possibly true I have to admit, as it used to be given to calm the violent and dangerous patients. It is however also an effective treatment for patients with deep clinical depression. Besides the patient having to agree and sign a consent form since the nineteen sixties, the treatment itself has been greatly modified. Every patient is examined physically by a doctor on admission, prior to being prescribed ECT, and before receiving it. Medication is given prior to the treatment to ensure only the minimum shock occurs. Just a flicker of a muscle is sufficient. Anaesthetic is a must since the fifties. Anaesthetist, doctor, and two or three nurses are needed to administer, assist and observe the patient recovery just as in any other operation. The most staggering miracle performed through ECT that I witnessed was in Amberstone. A catatonic man in his forties was admitted on a Friday. He had had a series of traumas precipitating his illness and the need for admission. He was mute when he was admitted; he had not been eating nor sleeping for several weeks and was in a sorry state. He was just staring into space. The consultant prescribed a series of 6 ECTs to start the next day, a Saturday. This was rare: ECT used to be given over three weeks, at a rate of two a week, Tuesdays and Fridays. An anaesthetist had to be found in Eastbourne and everything was set up. The man had to fast overnight but I am certain this was no hardship to him.

I was off that weekend. When I came back on Monday I could not believe my eyes. There he was, sitting up in bed, eating his breakfast, and he greeted me cheerfully, smiling. He recovered fully within the next few weeks and was able to get back to his life.

Another ECT occasion I recall is in Park House in the late seventies. It was often given to outpatients then, they stayed from 9am to 4pm, or in some cases just till lunch-time if a relative could take them home. I was upstairs in the dormitory, where ECT were performed, watching over this gentleman who had come for his first treatment, waiting for him to recover. He had just opened his eyes when a little fat lady streaked in screaming wildly. He looked again and, with wide eyes and a beaming smile, said: 'Blimey, I did not know they provided this on the NHS!' He was better already!

One elderly man, an outpatient as well, suffering from depression, was found to be extremely constipated on arrival for his first session of ECT. The doctor decided to suspend the ECT and prescribed an enema forthwith… This was very productive; the chap was so relieved and surprised to be so, he offered us money for our pains, or for the relief of his own! (Don't worry we would not have dreamt of taking it!) He did not need ECT after all; instead we gave him all kinds of good dietary advice to go home with.

Another morning another of our patients walked in, and, just as she would have asked for a cup of tea, demanded an ECT straightaway as she did not feel well. In the past she had recovered from a severe bout of depression with this treatment, her experience was positive, certainly. But that day all she needed was to talk about whatever was on her mind, and this was enough to help.

ECT, like anti-depressants, is only effective when people are depressed clinically. It will not work for existential depression, being fed up or miserable.

Earlier on I did touch on the fact that brain surgery stopped being performed at Hellingly by the sixties. However research were still being done in that area as, possibly in the late sixties, a new laser treatment was discovered; revolutionary, Itrium Implant was hailed as the miracle cure for intractable depression on a BBC documentary of the time. The criteria for referral for this very costly treatment to the Maudsley Hospital were very strict. The patient's illness had to be obdurate, of some duration and the patient or the relatives had to consent. Then the patient was assessed at the Maudsley for suitability. R. had had an Itrium Implant seven years before she joined us. A very bright and educated woman (she told me she had been taught by Margaret Thatcher!) she had a fantastic sense of humour and a caustic wit, often spiteful, which often took us by surprise. However she felt depressed, had no taste for life and no interest in anything. She had for this reason given up a prestigious job as a journalist in London and now lived with her parents. She begged to be referred again for another IT as she believed the previous one had made such a difference in her life… for at least 6 years anyway. Though the consensus of opinions was fairly negative as to her prognosis she did manage to get the treatment. But this was not the miracle cure she expected. She stayed on our books until she reached 65 then was transferred to the team for the Elderly Mentally Ill at the Conquest Hospital in the eighties.

Tender loving care, TLC, was the by-word in the seventies. "Support" was a necessary thing; unfortunately it became unmentionable by the late eighties. (In 2000 the then Chief Executive in Hastings told us we did not do "maintenance"…

He was right but what does this say about Mental Health Services?)

So let me tell you a story about TLC. In Camber ward was a patient diagnosed with schizophrenia, who was completely unmanageable. She was huge and loud, violent and unpredictable, no medication could touch her; most patients and staff feared her. Dr Johnston told me once she would not attack you if you did not show fear...This is as may be, but if someone comes towards your stomach with their fist and shows a menacing face, believe me, it is hard to look nonchalant! Another example of her behaviour was one lunch-time when she started shouting obscenities at the top of her voice in the dining room, throwing the plate of food she had in her hand to the other side of the room. Imagine what it was like for the other patients, most of them riddled with anxiety! Enough to give anybody indigestion, or cut your appetite altogether!

One day during a ward round her management was discussed at length, as usual. Ideas were floated as what could be done to help. Nancy A, a lively, warm, jolly, mothering Social Worker, proposed to see that patient on a one-to-one basis an hour every day. Most of us would have balked just at the idea. I thought she was very brave. And then slowly, little by little, we started noticing the changes in Sheila's behaviour. She was becoming more and more approachable, and even amenable. The funniest thing is that she began to speak with Nancy's well modulated tones and refined words. It was remarkable. Sheila was able eventually to be discharged home, to her husband and children, with medication, and visited by Nancy and Community Nurses for several months. She never came back as an in patient. I heard in 2003 through the grapevine that she had died of cancer.

Occupational therapies, formal or otherwise, were an essential part of patients' recovery. Activities with comradeship and a positive atmosphere provide equal and friendly rapport between staff and patients, all conducive to increased self-worth and self-confidence. There was an array of these activities to choose from.

To start with patients attended the OT department where, besides the proverbial cuddly toys and weaving baskets or tray making, they were assessed for other interests according to their needs. They could chose knitting or sewing, painting, mosaic and all kinds of other creative work. In the afternoons social games were played, which facilitated interaction, self-confidence and fun. When the department was closed, on Wednesday afternoons or weekends nurses would organise activities themselves, go for walks or chat with the patients. Coach trips were organised in the summer. It was funny to watch the weary looking patients appearing very much as though they were on their way to the scaffold, being coaxed or jollied along onto the coach by the staff. Then a few hours later you would see them back, cheerful, lively, chatty, obviously having had a great time.

If patients preferred, they could opt for other activities such as work in Industrial Therapy (for a little money), Park House greenhouse, the gardens, the farm, the printing shop etc. etc. for work rehabilitation.

When in charge of the Day-Patients it was part of my job to visit them in their various places of work. I enjoyed that. I was always welcome and the atmosphere was always convivial, staff and patients merging together. Charlie Kennett's woodwork shop was a hubbub of activity and deep debates.I always found the discussions, which Charlie often initiated, particularly stimulating and enjoyable. One morning we were debating whether it was good to get things off our chests and how this could be done. I said it would be great if we could go into a wood and have a really good scream sometimes. There was a newcomer in the workshop that day. He did not look depressed or anxious, with reasonable eye contact. He was pleasant, sociable, well turned out, clean and smart. I thought he could be a visitor. I was a bit puzzled by him. Anyway, in response to my remark, quietly he said: "My wife used to scream a lot". Then as it does happen, the conversation drifted off on to other subjects and I left. A few days later I asked Charlie who this man was. Well, he was a patient; he happened to have murdered his wife! I gave the place a miss for a few days after that...

I would like to share with you a bizarre recovery in Park House. Through the course of a day I frequently walked through the wards; I was familiar with most patients if only by sight. One very withdrawn lady who I had seen for several months in Camber dining room did not seem to progress. At lunch, she always sat staring at her full plate, or blankly into space and stayed there well after the other ladies had gone from the room. I kept saying "hello" but she never responded. One fine day I could not believe my eyes, she was actually eating her meal, her face made up, smiling at me, altogether a different person, she greeted me first and said "Hello!" I was so pleased to see this change in her, so staggered, that I had to pop into the office to ask the ward staff what was the miracle treatment she had received, the reason for this dramatic cure. They looked a bit blank, a bit sheepish even, and told me she had banged her head on a doorknob, getting up after a fall. Since then she had not looked back. Just imagine if anyone proposed this as a remedy on admission...

In the middle sixties different ranges of antidepressants, like MAOIs and Tricyclics came on the scene; then neuroleptic depot drugs like Depixol and Modecate in the early seventies. Given by injection at regular intervals, weekly, fortnightly, three weekly or monthly, (occasionally 5 or 6 weekly but then relapse is more likely to occur), these depot drugs are very effective in treating psychotic disorders. They allow many people to lead a reasonably normal life in the community, to hold a job and cope with a family.

MAOIs have lethal effects if taken with certain food: cheese, Marmite, yeast, some kind of beans, and many I have forgotten; this list increased over the years as each side-effect discovered was added to it. It was interesting to hear that bananas were back on the menu after it was found that the African Chief who had experienced the side effect was in the habit of eating bananas skin and all!

Powerful anti-depressants are rarely used today, due to the possibility of lethal overdoing. In the seventies, rather than using antidepressants some doctors preferred to use very small doses of Depixol injections to treat depression, or for behavioural problems. I did not personally think it was helpful. Moreover years later some doctors, when too pressed for time to be able to read chronic patients' thick files thoroughly, were likely to increase the dosage when the carers reported the patient to have relapsed. I believe they often jumped to the conclusion that these patients were schizophrenic as soon as they read that the patient had been prescribed "Depixol" in the past. Now let's not blame the doctors so much as the system: The time given to the patient has been reduced considerably over the years. Up to the early nineties I think, every first appointment with a psychiatrist was of an hour, now often three-quarters of an hour have to do. This is impossible. It reduces the interview to a series of set questions to the patient, a quick diagnosis and a giving of pills. For anybody not in the business you have to realise that in this time the doctor has to read the file, interview the patient, write his notes and dictate a letter to the GP. Patients always expect the old style of psychiatrist: not only to cure them of their affliction, but to be patient, understanding, and most of all to

90

listen to what they have to say. Those days are gone I am afraid; it is demoralising to Mental Health professionals, regulated by a thoughtless machine aiming to treat as many patients in the shorter possible time, with as few employees as possible. Bureaucracy has taken over to reduce cost and litigation.

Getting back to the seventies, a middle-aged patient I knew was diagnosed with "Monosymptomatic Delusional Psychosis"; in plain language she was deemed to have only one delusion: she believed her husband was unfaithful, and this distressed her very much. She was prescribed and given Depixol. Then we found out that her husband was indeed having an affair, right under our noses, with another of our patients…who made no secret of it. Despite informing our doctor of this important development, that our lady had no delusion, her belief was a fact, we were persuaded to go on with the treatment as it improved her symptoms. It made me very unhappy but I complied: medical opinion prevailed.

When a year later the same doctor asked me to double the dosage, as our patient was absolutely distraught that her husband had gone out on Christmas morning to visit his mistress and give her his present (…), I was livid myself. I did not manage to get this doctor to reconsider, nor did I get any joy from the consultant in charge, who supported his registrar. I refused to give this injection any more; I felt the dear lady was thoroughly brainwashed; she really thought she was mentally ill, she did not think she had the right to be jealous and thought she needed the increase in medication. I refused to collude with her husband by giving her the injection… A Community Psychiatric Nurse was asked to visit her at home and administer it… It still upsets me.

A few of our patients, mostly young women, had personality problems no medication could change. Many were going through

91

prolonged adolescence. More helpful were psychological methods, or talking therapies. One young lady about 20 years old had us running around in circles, taking overdoses, cutting her wrists, getting up to all sorts. She was prescribed all kinds of medication to use and abuse. Eventually she grew out of this and did not need us any more. I hope we helped in the process. I met her some twenty years later in Lewes. She recognised me straightaway. She presented her husband who was with her; she was obviously as pleased to see me as I was to see her, and she made this heart-warming remark: 'We do get better you see!'

From 1973 psychologists were allocated to wards, participated in team meetings and ran therapy groups. (I co-facilitated a Social Skills group with Christine Raafat when the Day Service was up and running). Nurses and social workers were keen to learn methods to enable patients to recover with or without medication. We were greatly encouraged by the then nursing management to pursue training in these therapies in the hospital setting or in different locations. We came back from these courses to share and discuss our new knowledge with our colleagues. Books seemed to materialise everywhere for our enlightenment; my first discovery in a second hand bookshop was Fritz Perls "Gestalt Therapy Verbatim", a revelation. I read anything I could get on the subject of helping others, and I helped myself by the way. So enthusiastic was I that I must have bored many, as I talked about what I had just read to anyone who would listen. A friend said about me at the time: "Ah! Elisabeth's new book!"

Doctors, psychologists, and others gave symposiums at Woodside for us all. Unfortunately most ward nurses could not attend as these happened between 12.30 and 2pm, when they had to hand over to the other shift, besides serving meals. Working with Day-Patients allowed me to attend during my lunch breaks. It was fascinating to listen to these learned professionals from various disciplines discuss cases, and offer very different opinions and alternatives therapy methods. I was amazed to discover there that nurses were considered a nuisance by some of these people. It was envisaged once it would be great to dispense with us altogether, when technology was such that robots and gadgets could fulfill our role in every way, clinical procedures, distribute medication, food etc... They were all getting carried away with the idea. The only nurse in the room, I was appalled by the perverse enjoyement of their Orwellian vision. I could not believe these supposedly intelligent professionals, with academic learning and sophisticated training in psychology, could be so lacking in the basic introspection to realise how petty they sounded. Then our Dr P brought everything back to sanity by carrying the idea to a pitch... Order was restored.... Indeed I learnt a lot in those seminars... I was quite shocked by a case conference another time, concerning a young anorexic girl. It was made clear that it was the unhappy and twisted mother who had, unconsciously over the years used food as a weapon, or a poison, to get back to her family she professed to love and care for. She, who made sure she was slim, had cooked and cooked and fattened them all up, apart from our patient who had resisted by becoming anorexic. I found this story horrific. Don't you?

The medication available, Depot injections, Lithium therapy and modern anti-depressants, facilitated patients improving and being discharged much earlier than they would have in the past but at the same time referrals went up. People seemed to be more agreeable to being admitted than they had been in the past; indeed some would do anything to be in hospital.

In 1973 three Senior nurses were sent to Chiswick Polytechnic to train in Community Nursing, Juliette Lusted, Nan Carr and

Derek Budd. They were to become Hellingly Hospital's first Community Psychiatric Nurses. Juliette, based in Park House, worked for the Hastings area; soon others joined her to form a team with John Manghan as a nursing officer; J.P P, Ron Crouch, Peggy Knowles, Simon M, Ted W, et al. They initially visited people in their homes after discharge to follow their progress. It was not long before GPs started referring patients to these CPNs to prevent admission.

Other patients were asked to attend Park House as outpatients for one to three days a week, to attend OT and be seen by a doctor if any problems occurred. Voluntary Transport, organised by the Royal East Sussex Hospital, was provided from their home in Hastings and Rother. In-patients using ward facilities tended to take priority in the ward and out-patients could be neglected. As I was working through the two shifts I was more in a position to be involved with the Day-Patients than other staff; I made it my business to find out how they were and report any problems to the Charge Nurses for the doctor's attention. I recall one occasion when I noticed a young woman I had not seen before in the sitting room on her own, looking vague and withdrawn. I wondered why she was not in Occupational Therapy where most people were supposed to be. It turned out she was not a patient at all! She had wandered in, from Hailsham, and just wanted some peace.

THE DAY-PATIENTS DEPARTMENT.
1973-1982

Back at Hellingly from May 1972, after the break-up of my marriage, in part-time work, I felt a bit of a square peg due to my unusual working hours, without the opportunity to get on in my career either. So I was thrilled when in 1973 Bryan Thorne, Senior Nursing Officer, meeting me in a corridor, asked me if I would be interested to take the day-patients under my wing as my working hours suited theirs. This was right up my sleeve. He gave me more or less carte blanche in the setting up of this new service. For a little while I was given one Camber' side rooms as my office, with the support of Jean-Pierre Parmainteny, the Charge Nurse at the time. After a few weeks, the system working to everyone's satisfaction, referrals coming thick and fast, the Day-Patients "situation" (as Mr T. used to call our set-up) moved to the West front of Park House. We had a large sitting room for the patients, a large office/ clinic with a little room at the back; this used to be the barber's room years before and the paraphernalia was still there.

Our day-patients, who had initially mixed with the in-patients for lunch, very soon branched out to form their own group. Our Rose, a motherly and stalwart character, took the lead and assembled two tables together so that they could be by themselves. I was quite chuffed that they had initiated this move. We were now a cohesive unit.

Tentatively and increasingly around then, depending on my confidence, I started to wear mufti; first I replaced my uniform with a blue dress buttoned at the front with pockets; it was very close to a uniform without the rigidity of a starched collar and cuffs. It made me aware how the uniform had been a protection, shielding my shyness. Mr Thorne noticed this absence of uniform one day: he approved but recommended I should wear a name badge. The wards soon followed suit. For a while we had what I called a fashion competition amongst the women, it was a bit ridiculous I seem to remember, but everyone calmed down eventually.

Helen Dalton, SEN, was allocated to work with me sometime in 1975 and a year or so later, Sally Fox, who was still an auxiliary nurse then.

My demands to the wards for their doctor eventually bore fruit: Dr Salama joined us, and we did not have to share him with other wards. Always courteous, calm and efficient, he was a learned physician but also a friend. He was kind and fun to work with. He was with us a couple of years. He was then allocated to another ward and not long afterwards became clinically depressed following relationship entanglements. In '76, that hot summer of 76, in August, he disappeared from Amberstone where he was being treated and was found dead several weeks later in Park woods; he had given himself an intravenous injection of Insulin…

He came to see us not long before he disappeared. We had a little chat and on leaving he took my hand, with my bunch of keys in it, and gave it a squeeze saying goodbye; the look on his face I now read as desperate… Helen has a note from him, dated 14th August thanking her for the postcard from Berlin. He stated he was home and looking forward to seeing us soon…

Also in 1976, I applied for the advertised job of Sister in charge of Day-Patients, the post I had held as a Staff Nurse. Mr Rheinholds, who interviewed me, along with Bryan Thorne, made it a condition that my eldest son would not walk to Park House on his return from school but straight home. It so happened that his son and mine made their way back to the hospital from the primary school at Hellingly village, then played together in the area surrounding Park House for half an hour, waiting for me to come out of work. Mr R. did not think it was appropriate. I was quietly miffed about this, but I had to agree of course. I was not that keen on my son being a latchkey kid, but there you are…

The consultants' rounds were invaluable in the learning process. They could be of two to four hours' duration. In the wards as many staff as possible participated. Each patient' case would be analysed and discussed in as much depth as it was necessary; family history, background, psychological profile, presentation, problems, medication, therapeutic approaches, etc. Finally the patient was seen, again at some length, to listen to their views, hopes and expectations, and arrive at a suitable treatment programme with their agreement. These meetings could be nerve-wracking for some patients, certainly. A few found it impossible to speak if they were particularly anxious. I was present once in Camber when Dr Pendlebury surprised us all, he made all of the staff go out in order to enable the patient to relax and say what she wanted to say.
(Nowadays, in the Community, meetings relating to patients usually also last a whole morning. However they are not to discuss cases but to decide which member of the team will take on the patient on his/her case load, with a short letter from the GP for information if they are lucky.)

These weekly rounds were a little easier in our department as the patients were familiar with us all and we were never more than four in the room. The staff consisted of the consultant, (Dr P or Dr B), the registrar, Helen or Sally and me.
One of our Day-Patients had never been able to cope with the loss of her husband who had died several years before. She constantly demanded different medication, which she did not

take. (I was often concerned, visiting patients, how often their cupboards were chucker-block with bottles full of potentially dangerous medication) She regularly terrified her grown up children with threats of suicide if they did not come every time she called them.

She found it difficult to get any interest in anything other than her bodily symptoms. When I had to announce to our patients that C, a man who had gone out of his way to help everyone, and especially her, as she had expected him to drive her here, there and everywhere, had suddenly died of a heart attack, she responded by saying she had a stomach-ache and could we do something about it. I was quite shocked with her callousness at the time.

We did not know how to help this lady; we asked Dr P to see her and review her management. When she came in she told him she could not bear it any longer and was going to kill herself. He asked how. She replied by putting her head in the oven (gas was still toxic by the way). He explained at some length, in the soft-spoken, slow, measured words of his, with his deep voice, how to make sure this would work: first she had to choose a time she did not expect anyone to call, then to draught proof all doors and windows, on and on he went, and the rest of us listened in amazement. She eventually cut him short by shouting at us:

"He is a doctor and he is telling me to kill myself!"

"No, you told me that is what you wanted to do" said Dr P.

"What about my daughters?"

"What about your daughters?"

"I could not do that to them!" then furious she turned to us (we were agog) as witnesses: "Listen to him, a doctor, and he is telling me to kill myself!"

"No, you were telling me you wanted to kill yourself, I was just telling you the best way to do it...."

In a few minutes he had taken her through the scenario and had turned the situation around.

I often thought it was good to work with both Dr B and Dr P as we did. They were opposite in every way. They saw everything differently but Dr P. was my Guru. He took his time with the patients, analysed everything and nothing seemed to shock or surprise him. I often thought that if you told him you had killed someone he would not turn a hair. He seemed to understand every human frailty, the why and wherefore, and he tried to help me to be more understanding too. I was ranting about someone to him once, furious at whatever that person had said or done. He could not calm me down; I told him that I was fed up understanding her, what about me being understood for a change? (That irritated him I could see.) There is no doubt he was a great influence in my life. For years afterwards when I was in a fix I used to imagine what he would say about the situation and I usually came up with a sensible answer to my problems.

I accused him of being cynical once, he replied he was a realist; it comes to many of us eventually… Dr P., if I remember correctly, had been part of an amateur dramatic group in Cambridge or Oxford. Not surprisingly he used his voice to great effect. He could speak so softly you had to listen attentively; he could bellow with laughter or with fury. Strangely enough he never frightened me. Something had angered him in the ward once and he caught me in the corridor to ventilate about it, he was like a roaring lion; I watched him fascinated, and made a terrified face with my hands shaking in the air to calm him down, and he did, straightaway, with a laugh.

He always took his time with everyone. He gave you time. He listened more than he talked, there could be long silences in his interviews, often he unnerved people who complained afterwards that he never said anything; silence allows the

99

patient to open up. I occasionally wondered whether he was quiet because he was at a loss as what to say; but there again when you have nothing to say it is better to say nothing. I am still practising!

Every one of his rounds was an education. I was going through some difficult times at home and I remember a particular discourse he gave us about a patient who carried her cross. It made me take stock and helped me change my situation.

Many of us working with him collected his catchy turn of phrases. They still pop out of our mouths at appropriate moments, its uncanny! He loved to shock the gallery. We were always a captive and mesmerised audience in our Day Unit. We glanced at each other, Helen, Sally and I, when he made one of his stupefying reflections, and giggled madly about it as soon as he had gone. I was telling him once that one of our ladies, an elderly widow, had a recurring eye problem: "Aaah…the eye….the vagina of the mind…" he said. Personally I prefer "window to the soul", even if a cliché! Several months later I took a day off when we expected him for his round as I had an eye infection… I did not want him to extrapolate about me!

As for Dr B he did not beat about the bush. He was outgoing, forceful, dynamic, business-like, not into analysis. His rounds were short and sharp; a bit like a whirlwind clearing the cobwebs. What's the problem? Let's see what we can do about it; we have a medication of choice for you… He gave everyone, including the staff, instant hope. He could be great fun as well, very witty. One young woman suddenly developed hysterical blindness (sorry reader if I offend you with these non PC words by the way). She started wearing dark glasses and used a white stick. We were telling Dr Bott how, despite this handicap, she managed to produce beautiful embroidery in OT, using harmonious colours, following the designs to perfection. Quick as a flash he said "Wave a fiver in front of her and see what she does!" We liked the idea; we did not put it to the test…

A lovely and warm–hearted Indian lady doctor replaced Dr Salama for a short while, and then Dr Johnston joined the team until we moved to Hastings.

Dr Margaret Ann Johnston, or Ann, as she preferred to be called, joined us when she must have been in her early fifties. She was an extraordinary woman. Everyone now remembers her as "the lady doctor in a wheel chair". I would like to say a bit more about her as we became friends, and she made a big impression on me.

She contracted polio when she was pregnant with her first child. She had been working with poliomyelitis patients without being vaccinated herself. Formidable as well as indomitable, fully paralysed for several months, with sheer will power, determined to regain the use of her independence, from being fed by drip she was eventually able to use the upper half of her body. She had to use a wheelchair for the rest of her life but managed to bring five children into the world, and bring them up, all healthy and bright.

I am told that she and her family moved into the flat which used to be at the back of Park House for a short while when they came to Sussex, before moving to Horam. By the time we knew her she worked full time, driving to work everyday in her mini traveller; (My ten-year-old son thought she came all the way down the road from home in her wheelchair!). She travelled all over the world, notably to Australia, to visit her eldest daughter and family.

She lived on her own after the children left and her husband died. We did not usually worry too much about her as we knew she had help in the neighbourhood, but one day she had not arrived by 10am; I think it had snowed, it was a bitter winter's day anyway, and we were a bit concerned, so I decided to drive up the road to see if anything was amiss. I found her in her garage, sitting on the ground by her mini. She had fallen down as her chair slipped away when she was trying to sit in the car. I could have cried to see her there, so valiant and uncomplaining, smiling and pleased to see me. I often wished she could have a good moan!

At work she was greatly admired and loved by many. She seemed to know every patient in Park House, spent time with everyone, stopped in the corridors for chats, held hands, comforted and empathised. She came back from the ward once telling us that one of the ladies had stopped her to warn her there were men under the floor; "No dear, there are no men there" she said, trying to reassure her. Well, as she uttered these words, two men emerged from a hole in the floorboards.. They

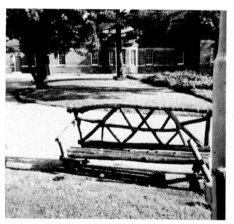

The little rustic bench in front of Park House...it was removed in the late seventies.

had been repairing the central heating.

She could be strict and impatient at times with what she saw as foolish behaviour. She slapped my bottom once, quite forcefully in what was supposed to be mock anger: I must have said something that had annoyed her. This surprised me but made me laugh. We did have a kind of mother/daughter relationship it must be said.

She could be the iron hand in the velvet glove; once she had made her mind up no one could budge her; she did not give way to emotional blackmail from the patients either. A woman who had had several admissions to dry her out from alcohol threatened to kill herself if she was not readmitted. Ann stuck to her guns; she told her to seek help from AA and would not give in. I was worried about this myself, but Dr Johnson was proved right. Admission would have been more than useless in the long run. It takes guts to give the "therapeutic thump". (This formula from Nancy A. I never forgot: you tell the truth as you see it). Most people respect integrity. In those days we were expected to be real, direct and genuine to enable possibility of change of behaviour. Of course we do not always get the response we hope for. For instance when Anne told one of our very bright patients (the lady who had the Itrium Implant in fact) who complained she was unable to do something, that of course she could, if she wanted to, and that lady replied spitefully: "In that case you walk"…

When Anne retired we kept in touch at least once a year around Christmas; she liked to know how everyone was getting on. We last spoke together in November 2002, when she told me she was moving to live with her daughter Allison and the family in the New Forest. She was to let me know her address when she got there. I was still waiting when exactly a year later I found out she had just died. It turns out she had not moved until September or October 03, after all.

From 1975 every year the Community staff was told to prepare for the move to Hastings the following year. This was to be the first stage of the hospital closure. I worried over this, as my children were too young to be left on their own for any length of time. I wanted very much to continue my work with the Day Patients; I was eager to see how we could develop it but I was not that keen to move. My children were settled, they used the hospital crèche until they started primary school at Hellingly village. The crèche did not cater for school aged children but, just in time for me, the holiday club was initiated and run voluntarily on a kind of rota system by the parents for a year or so, in the ground floor of one of the first villas vacated, on the left at the top of the Drive. The following summer holiday a small prefab building with space for a playground was allocated for this purpose, and staff employed by the hospital to run the play-groups.

Around then I started to work voluntarily every Tuesday evening in Hastings with Helen Dalton and a nice little band of ex-patients who were keen on setting up a Day Centre for the MIND Charity . This was great fun! We cleaned and sanded down, painted and decorated a little room in Emmanuel church in Hastings for several weeks. Other staff occasionally joined us when we had a party, for instance for the opening and at Christmas. These evenings had been so popular that it was decided we would continue to meet weekly for an evening social club. It ran for a year or two until Helen left.

The Day Centre finally opened around 1980. Sally went to Hastings on a regular basis for quite a while to to guide the voluntary leader. The idea was for the patients to contribute to the running of the place in a democratic fashion, but it did not work out that way for very long.

Finally, in November 1982, a year after the Community Psychiatric Nurses, Sally and I left the hospital to run the new Day-Unit in the Community at Holmesdale House, in Hastings. I also took over the Depot Clinic from Mary Jo who had been running it one evening a week for several years at the Royal East Sussex Hospital.

It had taken seven years of preparation, planning and meetings to set up the Community team out there. Another stage of my working life had begun. This could be another story to tell, maybe...

Hellingly Hospital closed in the middle eighties. It has been empty since but for some of the surrounding buildings were sold off or are now used as administrative offices. The Crèche is still functioning.

Security guards and high metal fences did not stop vandals over the years from wrecking the place, breaking windows, getting in and setting fire to the clock tower in 2003; and, just a few months later, the then still active Social Club prefab building was gutted by fire, only days after our reunion to commemorate its forty years along with the hospital hundredth.

It is heartbreaking to walk around this vast dead hospital, this dead world, as it is but a shell full of ghosts; for each of us who worked there these ghosts may be only slightly different. Mine are of friends, of people I liked, and others too, who impressed me with their strong personalities or peculiarities, and let's not forget this other ghost, the one of this young wide-eyed hopeful girl who was me then… Voices, noises off, come to my mind, and it is nostalgic indeed.

AFTERWORD

9 October 2004

Latest plans for the brown site Hellingly Hospital seem encouraging to me. Last night four people employed by the property developers came to a meeting of Hellingly Community Park Trust to present their plans for future developments. The accent was particularly on the protection of the local wild life, the flora and fauna, badgers, owls, bats, dormice, voles, trees etc... They were at pains to show how sensitive they were to the keep the positive aspects of the surroundings; I even seem to remember someone mentioning aiming to keep the spirit of the place.

I was interested to notice some buildings would be designated to house bats under the roofs. I could not help smiling as someone worried that, with the new inhabitants, cats would start proliferating in the area and endanger the protected wild life. And this, after the descendants of Sr White's cats have apparently been eradicated!

Though it is a shame that our local landmark, the water tower, will have to go, as we were told it was so dilapidated nothing could be made of it, we were given to understand that some of the main building would be used in the structure of the new community.

Yes, I was encouraged to think life would breathe again on the site that was Hellingly Hospital.

AUTHOR'S CONTACT DETAILS

If you wish to get in touch with the Author please
email to:-

elisabethgimblett@tiscali.co.uk

_or_

editor@moonflowerbooks.com

Heading your message :- Elisabeth Gimblett